The GP's Guide to Personal Development Plans

Second edition

Amar Rughani

General Practitioner, Sheffield
GP Tutor for CPD, University of Sheffield

Forewords by

David Haslam
Pat Lane
and
Mike Pringle

Radcliffe Medical Press

© 2001 Amar Rughani

Radcliffe Medical Press Ltd
18 Marcham Road, Abingdon, Oxon OX14 1AA

First edition 2000

Reprinted 2001
Reprinted 2002

British Library Cataloguing in Publication Data

A catalogue record for this book is available from the British Library.

ISBN 1 85775 509 X

Typeset by Joshua Associates Ltd, Oxford
Printed and bound by TJ International Ltd, Padstow, Cornwall

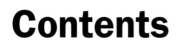

Contents

Foreword

The more everything changes, the more it stays the same. It is understandable that so many GPs feel overwhelmed by the apparently insurmountable opportunities that face them each and every day. There are constant exhortations to do more of this, that and everything else whilst nothing ever gets taken away. Along with the challenges come the concepts of clinical governance, appraisal, Revalidation, and personal and practice development plans. It is quite enough for many of us to bury our heads and wait for it all to go away.

For the great majority of GPs and practices, the concept of PDPs can seem totally underwhelming. But the simple fact is that PDPs are simply a concept that helps us do what we have always wanted to do–learn effectively, spot our weaknesses before they become problems, and increase our personal satisfaction.

This splendid book is readable, reliable and relevant. Amar Rughani shows that PDPs need not be a source of anxiety, but instead offers us a way to build our skills to help us all find a way through the contemporary difficulties of general practice.

And that is certainly something we all need.

Dr David Haslam
Visiting Professor in Primary Health Care, de Montfort University, Leicester
Chairman Elect, Royal College of General Practitioners
May 2001

Foreword

General practice is undergoing an unprecedented cultural change and traditional medical school education followed by postgraduate training has not adequately prepared many doctors for the challenges they now face. The concepts of lifelong learning, clinical governance and Revalidation are difficult to assimilate for the hard-pressed general practitioner. Patients expect doctors to deliver value, integrity and equity. The key to meeting these demands lies within education and training.

Most GPs resent the introduction of the Postgraduate Education Allowance (PGEA) system introduced in 1991. They have found the accumulation of certificates of attendance at meetings to be a frustrating chore, open to abuse, and yielding little professional satisfaction. A significant number of GPs have preferred to conduct their professional development through personal learning plans and portfolios that are mentored and peer referenced. Most practices conduct 'team'-based learning events to assist collaboration and consistency within primary healthcare, and the GP tutors have been prime movers in stimulating and developing this process.

Throughout the North Trent Network, GP tutors have encouraged fellow GPs to consider moving away from the concept of accredited meetings to a system of accredited learning. In April 2001, over 50% of GPs in South Yorkshire and South Humber were earning their PGEA through portfolios.

It makes sense to use the personal development plan to:

- earn the PGEA
- inform Revalidation
- contribute to practice professional development plans and clinical governance
- provide a reflective record of achievement and future learning needs.

This GP's guide to personal development plans is both timely and functional. It is written by a full-time GP who has an excellent understanding of the hopes and concerns of his colleagues from all types of practice. The guide has the potential to usefully assist all GPs to demonstrate true professionalism for 'external' agencies that seek proof of quality. We are all capable of improvement and the chapters in this book give us the tools with clarity and purpose. The inclusion of assessment guidelines in this second edition will contribute to the quality assurance of PDPs in a transparent and formative manner among GP tutors and their colleagues in general practice.

The production of PDPs by all doctors is expected from April 2001. It is time to engage in this process by sharing your concerns and aspirations with your local GP and primary care tutors. The culture is already moving to incorporate the ethos of protected time for learning and Amar Rughani's book should prove to be an important catalyst to effect this change.

Dr Pat Lane
Director of Postgraduate General Practice Education
Sheffield
May 2001

Foreword

Most innovations are taken up by a small group of GPs. They are then taken up by 'early adopters'. Only then is a new way of working ready to be taken up by the majority of the profession. Computerisation is a classic case study and only now, with wide uptake, is an element of compulsion creeping in.

Continuing professional development (CPD) has no such pedigree. While the shortcomings of continuing medical education (CME) are widely acknowledged and the putative virtues of CPD are 'self-apparent', CPD has not even entered the 'early adopters' phase. The vast majority of GPs do not know another GP who is doing it.

Yet, we are all doing it. Much of CPD is the recognition of the learning we already do. Few innovations in my practice have come from attendance at a lecture – the traditional form of CME. Most have come from significant event auditing, reflection on our care and responding to uncertainty with an attempt to find an answer.

Although CPD is therefore being introduced without a platform of successful users, it is the system that is new, not the concepts. All GPs need help in seeing what it is and how they can do it, and the essential tool for this is a personal development plan.

This book is a clear and accurate statement – in language that we all can follow – of the whys and wherefores of personal development plans. It is an invaluable source of inspiration, information and education. I recommend it to all GPs.

Professor Mike Pringle
Chairman of Council
Royal College of General Practitioners
February 2000

Preface to the second edition

At the time that the first edition of this book was written, personal development plans (PDPs) were being advocated by the GP professional and regulatory bodies as an alternative to lecture-based CME. In several reports, their importance as a probable requirement for Revalidation was emphasised rather more than their educational potential but despite this less-than-ideal introduction, PDPs have been welcomed by many of the doctors who have used them. The reasons for this reflect the nature of adult learning. GPs have appreciated the opportunity to set their educational agenda, to be accredited for the learning that arises naturally from the workplace, and to choose educational activities that reflect their needs and learning styles. Tutors have developed stronger links with their colleagues and have used PDP meetings as an opportunity to provide mentorship, and to encourage the sharing of ideas and support between practitioners.

This communal activity has meant that much experience has been gained about how PDPs work at a practical level, and important lessons about the areas with which learners have difficulty and the ways in which the plan can be used to encourage the development of the individual have been learned. In this edition, I have used this experience to update the chapters on writing the development plan. In addition, I have added a new chapter on assessing PDPs that uses an interactive approach to help readers develop the content and mechanism of their plans year-on-year.

For those who have yet to write their first development plan, I believe that this book will provide a straightforward introduction and take the mystery out of the process. Additionally, for the growing number of doctors that have a PDP, I hope that the new edition will offer some ideas that will help to make future learning both more effective and more enjoyable.

Amar Rughani
May 2001

Preface

'May you live in interesting times', as the Chinese would say. Whether that is a curse or a blessing is open to debate, but there is no denying that these are indeed interesting times to be a general practitioner with changes in the profession and society being spurred on by the information revolution, changing expectations and the demand for increased accountability. Doctors may be forgiven for feeling that to survive in today's world they need to combine the caritas of Dr Finlay with the technical proficiency of *ER* and the management skills of Sir John Harvey-Jones!

Such a feat may be impossible to achieve, but successful adaptation to the future should not be beyond us. This transition depends on acquiring the necessary skills and developing the appropriate attitudes with which the needs of patients can be met and job satisfaction preserved. In other words, adaptation is inseparable from education.

Postgraduate GP education was originally driven by personal and professional expectations and more recently by the postgraduate education allowance (PGEA). In future, Revalidation will be the prime influence on GP education and will require doctors to demonstrate that they have engaged in educational activity that is appropriate to the needs of the individual and of the practice. This requirement can be met by using a personal development plan, and in this book I have used my perspective as a GP tutor, and more importantly as a full-time GP, to show how such a plan can be produced and used. In this task I have been greatly aided by the advice and support of GP tutors and advisers in the UK but particularly in the Trent region, whom I wish to thank. I would also like to thank my GP colleagues in Sheffield – if the final product is readable, it is mostly due to them!

Amar Rughani
February 2000

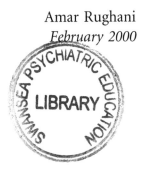

About the author

Amar Rughani is a GP in a large suburban practice in Sheffield and a GP tutor for continuing professional development at the University of Sheffield. His expertise in GP assessment derives from his work as an examiner for the RCGP and from personal experience of having completed Fellowship by Assessment of the RCGP. Using these perspectives, he is closely involved in developing a programme to help GPs come to terms with the future of postgraduate medical education and, hopefully, to enjoy the experience!

Acknowledgements

I would like to thank a few key individuals for the help they have given me. First and most importantly, my wife Sue for providing nurture whilst being neglected. Second, Dr Pat Lane for his constant enthusiasm and support. I would particularly like to thank my GP tutor colleagues, Nick Field, Mike Tomson and Arthur McFarlane, and acknowledge the debt that we owe to Dr Field for his pioneering work on portfolio learning.

I am also grateful to the following GPs for providing their wisdom: Steve Ball, Gary Chambers, Keith Collett, Diane Kelly, John Orchard, Mike Pringle, Linda Sykes, Chris Thorogood and Edward Warren.

For my children, Guy and Isabel

1 About learning

Key points

- Many GPs were never taught or shown how to learn.
- We need to think less about acquiring information and more about applying what we learn.
- Revalidation will require us to demonstrate our learning.
- Being able to admit our shortcomings is the first step to self-improvement.
- Time spent educating ourselves is as valuable as time spent treating patients.
- Most experiences can begin a learning cycle.
- Even before we create time, we must protect the time we currently have for reflection.
- We can study the changes we have made to our practice to determine how best to learn.
- Participating, evaluating and offering feedback all increase the value of educational opportunities.

Introduction

This handbook is about how GPs can determine their educational needs and address them through the use of 'personal development plans'. But surely, we've missed out a stage? Don't we need to establish first of all that there *is* a need to learn and that doctors are willing and able to engage in the process?

You may feel that such a need is obvious and therefore does not merit further discussion, but as a profession we are at a crossroads in many ways, not least with regard to how we equip ourselves for the educational demands of the future. The knowledge, skills and attitudes required for the rest of our professional lives may not be the same as those that many GPs acquired as students and in the early days of practice life. In addition, the pace of change seems overwhelming and many GPs are exhausted, apathetic or simply bewildered as to how to face the future. This is understandable, but one lesson from the past is that GPs are enormously adaptable, and seem able to resolve positive outcomes from competing demands.

So it could be with education. Although the demands to analyse our work, show improvements in patient care and root out the 'bad apples' in our midst feels like an imposition, it is probably the greatest opportunity we have had to focus our learning on what *we* think matters. The encouragement to learn from and help each other could lead to a change in culture in which GPs and their teams work together to bring about improvements in service and just as importantly, in job satisfaction.

So much for the rhetoric, but how exactly can this book help you? In this chapter we will consider the sort of people we are, how we have been taught to learn, how we currently learn, and how and why this will change in the future. I should point out that the observations in this chapter are made from a personal viewpoint.

Where have we come from?

This may seem to be a strange subheading but I'm interested here not so much in our social backgrounds as in the ways that we have been conditioned to learn

Let us consider why as GPs, our medical training places us at a disadvantage for our future learning.

Medical students are selected for, and succeed at, university partly on the basis of having very good powers of recall, a trait reinforced through the rituals of fact-based examinations and the exposure of ignorance on ward rounds. Acquiring knowledge is given priority, with those who are good at acquiring it being respected as peers and those who are good at imparting it being respected as teachers.

For the students of today, teaching has improved, but although more emphasis is given to the application of knowledge, teachers are still expected to *tell* students lots of things rather than to show them how to learn. In the past, students were not encouraged to question the assumption that factual knowledge was all-important or to challenge the usefulness of what they were taught. Even less were they given the opportunity to decide what they needed to know or to consider the importance of learning how to learn.

The way that we were brought up to be 'professionals' may also have impeded our learning. Our role models had many good points, but some were also authoritarian and gave the appearance of being self-sufficient and infallible. This influence coupled with the tendency as high-achievers to be poorly tolerant of the criticism of others, has made it hard for some to admit to themselves, let alone to others, that they have deficiencies which need addressing.

Where are we now?

These factors partly explain why, as GPs, we may behave in the following ways.

Learning in the traditional way

Resonating with the past, doctors like the familiarity of the postgraduate medical centre and the 'talk and chalk' sessions provided by experts who update our knowledge from their secondary care perspective. It seems fine, even pleasant when there is food and drink (we're only human after all) but the following questions are worth asking:

- How relevant is the subject-matter to general practice and indeed to our own practices?
- How much of it is just the old-fashioned information overload (theory) and how much of it addresses real problems in practice life (application)?
- To what extent are GPs involved in the session, either as providers or participants. If there is no GP resource, then the usefulness of such a session is likely to be much reduced.
- Learning should lead to a *change* in the way we do things, but how often is this our experience following such meetings?

Accruing knowledge is traditionally given a high priority. Interestingly, although we respect those peers who are well-informed, many GPs rate colleagues who display qualities such as caring, wisdom and enthusiasm even more highly. We know that education can fill gaps in our knowledge but may not realise that the learning process can also promote in us those attributes which we admire in others. For example, developing communication skills could help us to establish greater empathy with our patients, thus enhancing the 'caring' aspect of the doctor–patient relationship.

Choosing our educational activity

We often choose our education on the basis of what is on offer (and free) rather than because the topic is appropriate to our needs. When we do make an active choice we select our activity, such as attending meetings or even the articles that we read, in response to what we are interested in. This might seem quite reasonable, but the problem is that such an approach addresses what we *want* to learn rather than what we *need* to learn. Our interests, being personal preferences, tend to change with time, but our needs, because they represent deficiencies, will persist unless corrected by education.

Of course it is in no-one's interest for GPs to undertake educational activity which they need to do but have no desire to participate in, and the solution lies partly in getting doctors to define their needs and partly in providing education which stimulates and entertains.

We feel comfortable with being the passive recipients, i.e. in 'being educated', and may not like attending meetings in which participation is required in case our ignorance is exposed or our views shot down. However, when such meetings are made relevant to GPs by using a GP resource and encouraging non-threatening participation, they are often thought to be a success by those attending, many of whom see the advantage of this method of learning over the traditional lecture style.

Learning from experience

In our practices, experiences from which we can learn are ubiquitous, but there are barriers that prevent us from realising this learning potential. Self-sufficiency is one such barrier, impeding us from talking openly with our colleagues let alone with other members of the team. Another problem is that too much self-esteem may be bound up with the notion of infallibility. If we adopt this notion, perhaps because we think it is part of professionalism, it can make us dogmatic and inflexible, less likely to establish our needs and even less to respond to them. We may become concerned that making changes is like admitting that what we were doing before was wrong. It wasn't – it's just that what we choose to do now is better.

GPs also worry about personal factors. If we do admit a mistake or expose a weakness to a colleague, particularly a partner, how might they react? The risk of being made to feel inadequate, or worse still losing their respect, seems great, but deeply rooted though this fear is, it can be overcome by encouraging an atmosphere of openness with the promise of support rather than censure.

Examples given later in this book show how to achieve this. It is a point I emphasise because the benefits that such an environment can bring both in educational and personal terms are huge. It would be a shame to miss out!

Why should we move on?

Now for the sticks and carrots.

The postgraduate education allowance (PGEA) has been criticised because it is not based on our educational needs, does not encourage us to reflect on our work and learn from it, and shoehorns education into seemingly arbitrary categories. Its influence on our education will be diminished by the arrival of Revalidation, which will involve GPs in demonstrating that they are engaged in educational activity that consolidates good practice and demonstrates evidence of learning. The scheme being considered will require GPs to keep educational 'portfolios' of what they have done, what they have learned and how they have applied it. We will consider this in more detail in Chapter 3, but it is clear that being passively educated and going to meetings, which perhaps we learn nothing from, will no longer be appropriate.

Kenneth Calman, when Chief Medical Officer, gave a strong push to the creation of personal development plans for all professionals in the healthcare team, which took account of the needs of the practice as well as the individual. He called these 'practice professional development plans' (PPDPs) and the implication is that GPs will have to learn to use such plans and to integrate them with those of their colleagues.

What then of the carrots? No GP wants to be poorly performing and all want to provide good patient care while making sure that the time spent on education is relevant and useful. The changes proposed will promote this by acknowledging that much of the time spent thinking about patient care and how it can be improved upon, in addition to the time taken through implementing changes, is in fact time spent on education. This *time*, which may quickly add up to many hours, can in the future be accredited. In terms of attitudes, we may come to see that our everyday experiences have educational value which in itself could make us think about what we do in a deeper way.

By setting the educational agenda, we can decide to spend our time improving skills in areas which *we* feel will produce patient benefit. The skills needed may for example be identified from:

- Those interventions which are national or local priorities.
- The burden of disease or health problems in our area (e.g. Standardised Mortality Rates, teenage pregnancy rates).
- The interventions which we regard as being feasible for our practices.

Targeting education in this way may result in improvements in patient health which are visible at local level, thus reducing illness among the people we care for and so providing the motivation for us to continue our efforts.

Assessing our needs requires us to be honest with ourselves at the very least, and if we are able to involve others in this process, such as our partners and team members, then personal and team development are much enhanced. When people talk with and learn from each other, they feel valued and this has the effect of increasing confidence and esteem.

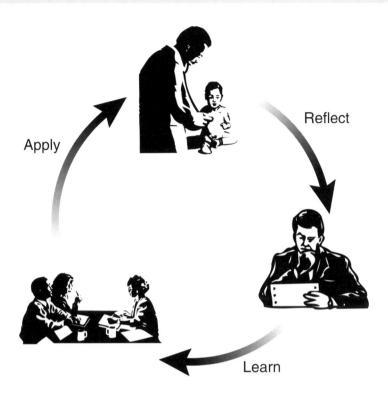

Figure 1.1 The learning cycle.

How can we move on?

In this section, we will first look at a model of how we learn, called the learning cycle, then use this as the basis from which to consider how improvements in our learning can take place, and finally comment on the time constraints with which we are faced.

The learning cycle (after Kolb)

This model demonstrates how experiences lead to a cycle of reflection and change which result in learning, as illustrated in Figure 1.1.

The doctor listens to the child's heart and hears a murmur, an *experience* which makes him uneasy and prompts him to *reflect* as to why this might be. The sense of unease alerts him to the fact that a gap exists between what he needs to know and what he actually knows. He realises that the cause of his discomfort is his inability to differentiate between an innocent murmur and a pathological one in a child of this age and he therefore defines his *educational need* as learning how to make this distinction.

In order to *learn*, he has to identify not only what he needs to learn but also how he wishes to address that need, and on the basis of this he decides to attend a course on community paediatric assessment. Having improved his skills, he is now able to *apply* his learning so that the next time he examines a child's heart and hears a murmur, he feels good because he is able to recognise it as being innocent, to reassure the parents and thus avoid causing distress through an unnecessary referral.

Figure 1.1 indicates that thinking about such experiences, putting them into context and considering their implications (the process of reflecting) allows us to learn from them and decide whether changes are needed. Changes are not always welcomed, but if they are regarded as improvements that *we* wish to make, then they are more likely to be put into effect.

We will now look more closely at three elements in the learning cycle: experience, reflection and learning.

Using our experiences effectively

The first thing is to recognise that *experiences* are the raw material from which we define our learning needs. All experiences have this potential, even the seemingly trivial ones and they are derived from:

- What we *do*: through consulting, treating patients, carrying out procedures, etc.
- What we become *aware of*: through reading, feedback, complaints, audit, analysis of data such as prescribing and practice activity (PACT), etc.
- What we *feel*: for example in response to significant events in our practice lives.

Although we could learn from *all* experiences, in reality some experiences highlight more important learning needs than others, a point which is considered in Chapter 2 on identifying and prioritising our learning needs.

Next, we need to raise our awareness so that we notice relevant experiences when they occur. Mostly, these experiences occur incidentally in our working lives and can therefore easily be lost unless they are recorded in a form such as a learning log.

In Chapter 6 on PUNS & DENS, we look at the use of one such log which is derived from the contacts we have with patients.

Learning to reflect

Thinking about our experiences allows us to reflect on those which make us feel uneasy and translate them into educational needs. This requires time which could be used more effectively if protected, and it is therefore useful to consider *when* we spend time reflecting. We recognise the importance of being free from interruption in our consultations, where we seek to avoid having our conscious thoughts interrupted, but the concept is just as important for periods of reflection when our subconscious minds are busy working.

A factor not often considered is that reflection is aided by being in a suitable environment. Hence *where* we do our thinking is important, and if a suitable place does not already exist, it is worth finding or creating an environment in which we feel relaxed enough to think about the implications of our experiences. Environmental influences often work in a Pavlovian manner such that being in favoured surroundings quickly helps to get us into the right frame of mind.

Making the most of our learning opportunities

We will consider this by looking at three areas: how as colleagues we can help each other, how we learn best and how to get the best value from the educational events we attend.

How can we help each other?

First, we should make sure that the *culture* of the practice is conducive to education. A good starting point is to look at the practice provision for study leave. Some doctors don't have this as a mutually agreed 'right', others don't take it for various reasons, including pressure of work, and some regard it as an extra few days of much-deserved holiday. It is important to regard time spent learning as being at least of equal value to time spent treating patients. While those who are delivering the service should avoid making absent partners feel guilty, those who are taking time out also need to recognise the value of feeding back what they have learned to those colleagues for whom it might be of interest.

Learning together means admitting that we have things to learn, or in other words that we have 'failings'. How then does this make us feel and what could we do to encourage the process and ensure that the experience is a positive one for those who take part in it?

Initially this may involve cultivating a relationship with a colleague, talking about work experiences, and sharing ideas and opinions. Later, as barriers break down and people start to talk about their deficiencies, this may take the form of actively listening and encouraging without being directive. The temptation to tell colleagues how *we* would do things should be resisted, and instead they should be encouraged to express *their* thoughts, what they see the problems as being and what strategies they can think of to address them. Those people who are thought to offer wise advice in fact rarely tend to give answers.

What are the best ways of learning?

The purpose of postgraduate education is to bring about improvements (i.e. changes) in the way we work. Therefore, it is worth cultivating those forms of learning which have led to changes in practice. Additionally, careful thought should be given to time spent on educational activities which consistently reap little reward.

The following exercise can help to make the distinction.

Think about three improvements that you have made to your clinical practice in the past three years. Write down what these changes are and the educational activities which prompted you to change.

Now consider how representative these activities are of the way you currently learn and ask yourself whether you should be engaging in them more often. For example, discussing a therapeutic advance using cases drawn from general practice might have been more persuasive in prompting change than learning about the same advance in a lecture.

We might well find that a proportion of the changes made were as a consequence of significant events in practice life. Recognising these as important influences for change might encourage us to use significant event analysis, as described in Chapter 7.

It is worth comparing our responses to this exercise with those of our colleagues. It may transpire that there are some forms of education that most people seem to gain benefit from and which could therefore be usefully encouraged. On this basis we might decide that clinical audit should be routinely conducted or that interactive meetings using facilitators could be arranged.

What about the educational events that we attend?

Practice-based learning is becoming more important, because it relates directly to our particular needs. However, much education will still be provided for GPs and there are steps that we can take to maximise the value of the events on offer.
These include:

- Attending events which address our needs and not attending those which don't.

- Playing an active part by contributing our perspective and insights, encouraging our colleagues to do likewise and questioning the relevance to GPs. These factors help to keep such events focused and useful.

- Asking 'Will this change the way I think or practice?' rather than just 'Did I enjoy the meeting?', as this gives a better idea of whether the educational event was a good use of our time. Hopefully, the two are not incompatible!

- Giving appropriate feedback to the course organisers. Evaluation sheets are getting better, and could include the following questions:
  - Were the objectives of the event achieved?
  - What did you learn?
  - In what way will your practice change as a result?
  - If the event was to be repeated, in what way could it be improved?

  Even if the forms do not ask these questions, trying to answer them and offering responses to those running the meeting is very useful. Most of the steps taken above should also apply to practice-based meetings, at which we could think about using evaluation forms for the reasons already mentioned.

Making more time for our learning

We've considered how to maximise the value of the time we currently spend learning, but where is *new* time to be found? In the past, educational activity was regarded as the individual's responsibility and finding time for it was a matter for the individual, but in the future, the practice will be asked to deliver on clinical targets such as coronary heart disease, depression and so on. To achieve this the practice will need to ensure that its members have the appropriate skills and knowledge, which means that education and finding the time to undertake it will become a practice concern.

Because there is a requirement to deliver on national targets, finding time for training is also a national responsibility. In some areas, funding has been made available for deputising cover to be provided where several practices close for a half-day of educational activity (the Doncaster TARGET scheme is a good example of this). Another more immediate possibility is that practices close during the day for a few hours of education at a time when patient demand may be a little less (e.g. midweek).

Patients could be advised well in advance that as a forward-looking practice, and in response to the demands of the public, time is being taken to improve the quality of care provided to them. This method may not suit all practices, particularly those with unusually high numbers of patient contacts. Different practices find their own ways of making time for education, so it is well worth asking colleagues what strategies they use, and seeing if they can be modified to suit your own circumstances.

Summary

GP education is now high on the political and public agenda. The changes proposed will require GPs to think more carefully about what they are learning and why, and to work with other colleagues and team members in achieving common goals. Far from being threatening, this will offer an opportunity to make education both more relevant and more enjoyable, an aim that can be achieved through planning what needs to be learned and reflecting on how useful that learning has been. But before such plans can be made we need to identify where our deficiencies lie and decide how we wish to prioritise them. This is the subject of the next chapter.

2 Identifying our learning needs

Introduction

Learning from our experiences

The methods of establishing our educational needs

Prioritising our learning needs

Summary

Key points

- Our needs are derived from a wide range of sources.
- Some sources are better suited to identifying particular needs than others.
- It is preferable to be familiar with a variety of techniques for establishing our needs.
- A number of agencies will have an influence on our educational priorities.
- We therefore need to set our priorities in consultation with others.
- A practical approach is to attend to safety first, then to national and local priorities.
- Most priorities will still arise from our personal agenda.

Introduction

In the previous chapter, we established the importance of basing our education on needs rather than wants and of using our experiences to initiate learning cycles. In

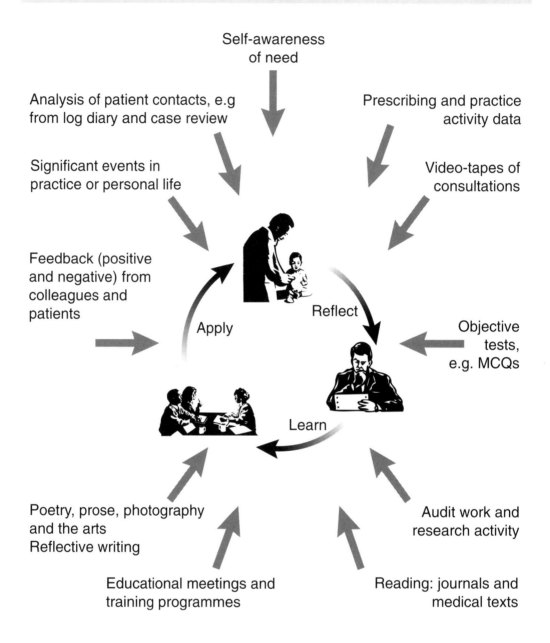

Figure 2.1 How GPs learn.

this chapter we will bring these themes together and consider where our experiences come from and how they can be used to identify deficiencies and therefore educational needs. Finally, we will consider the influences that make us prioritise some of these needs and not others.

Learning from our experiences

Figure 2.1, which has at its centre the learning cycle, was discussed in Chapter 1. The doctor examining the child has an experience, in this case a sense of unease derived from the physical examination, which leads on to a learning cycle. However, he could just as easily initiate learning cycles from other types of experiences drawn from the range of methods shown around him.

Each of these methods has the potential to make the doctor aware that he has a 'competence gap', which is a discrepancy between his current performance and the way he feels he would like to perform.

The methods of establishing our educational needs

Each of the methods shown in Figure 2.1 is discussed in more detail below. No one method is superior to the others, because in practice some methods are better suited to identifying certain needs compared with others. For instance, our communication skills with patients are probably better assessed through video-tape analysis of our surgeries than by questioning the patient about their satisfaction with the consultation.

In addition, not all methods will be available or be suitable. Not all practices, for example, will have the facility to use a camcorder in the consulting room, and very few practices are involved in research activity. Therefore to get a balance it is better not to rely on a single method, but to become familiar with the techniques that are feasible in your practice and use the appropriate ones according to the circumstances.

Self-awareness of need

Self-awareness, or using our opinion of our strengths and weaknesses in order to determine our educational needs, suffers from its lack of objectivity. Doctors have been shown to be poor at correctly identifying their deficiencies, but provided that we do not rely on this method alone and are honest with ourselves, self-awareness can be a powerful tool. Here are two exercises to help get self-awareness working for us:

- Imagine that you are in surgery and have just called your next patient. List the following:
  - the three types of problem with which you would feel most comfortable if presented
  - the three types of problem with which you would feel least comfortable if presented.
- Suppose that the time has come for the lines of responsibility within the practice to be redrawn and the doctors need to decide who among them is going to take a lead role with regard to important tasks such as business planning, nursing issues, team development and so on. List the following:
  - the three areas of responsibility with which you would feel most comfortable
  - the three areas of responsibility with which you would feel least comfortable.

Another approach is to ask:

- Which topics do I most enjoy learning about?
- Which topics do I least enjoy learning about?

Answering these questions with honesty allows us to reach more valid conclusions. We should think carefully about those areas that we find difficult and would prefer to avoid. Do these highlight educational needs, and if so do they need to be addressed as a matter of priority?

Significant events

Anything that is out of the ordinary in our personal or professional lives, and is significant either by its nature or because of its repercussions, is likely to be on our minds and has the potential to be learned from. Some might feel that significant events in our personal lives have little to do with our education, but this may not be the case.

Because events or experiences such as illness, bereavement or childbirth are personal, they affect us more deeply and therefore provide even greater potential for lessons to be learned. There must be many doctors who, for example having suffered grief in their own lives, find themselves better able to understand and manage the suffering of patients who have experienced a significant loss in theirs.

If *not* learned from, negative personal experiences may have deleterious effects on professional performance thereby demonstrating how closely personal and professional development are linked.

With regard to significant events in practice life, these can often be powerful motivators for change in our professional behaviour. Mostly, change occurs when negative (or critical) events occur, but there are also lessons to be learned from positive events.

The process of learning from significant events is called 'significant event analysis' and is discussed later in this book.

Feedback from colleagues and patients

Feedback from those we work with often comes in verbal form or from entries in patients' records, and for some doctors additional feedback is obtained through more formal systems such as case review or clinical audit. Patients may also provide feedback through avenues such as suggestions and complaints, by completing questionnaires or via patient participation groups.

Doctors do not manage their patients in isolation from their colleagues or indeed their patients, and feedback from them shows us what went well in addition to what might have been done better. Giving colleagues feedback on positive as well as negative events prevents an atmosphere of recrimination developing, and it is important when criticism *is* intended that it is delivered sensitively: 'Do as you would be done by' is a good approach.

No one enjoys being criticised and although feeling bad is a natural reaction and seems not to diminish with experience, ultimately there is satisfaction to be had in learning from our mistakes. When on the receiving end of criticism, after the initial flurry of denial has settled down, it is useful to ask ourselves whether, if faced with the same situation, we would act any differently. If the answer to this question is 'No', then either the criticism was not justified or our judgement is lacking. If the answer is 'Yes', then we have succeeded in identifying a learning need.

Video-tapes of consultations

There are certain barriers (including not having access to a camcorder!) to the use of this technique. The consulting room is considered to be the GP's inner sanctum, a private and secret place where observation may be unwelcome. In addition, few GPs believe that they consult poorly and so for some, the arguments for analysing the consultation may not be persuasive. However, the consultation is the cornerstone of general practice and no consultation is ever perfect.

Consultation analysis involves learning about a set of consultation skills that can be identified, taught, practised and incorporated in our own consultation style. The use of this approach has revolutionised the training of GPs and can help all of us to increase the effectiveness of our consultations and the satisfaction which both we and our patients experience. Although the mechanics of recording consultations is straightforward, feedback on consulting skills is a sensitive matter and needs to be given by someone who is trained for the purpose, such as a GP trainer. Discussion of consultation analysis is beyond the scope of this book, but as an introduction I would recommend the following short and very readable guide, written by a pioneer in this field: Tate P (2001) *The Doctor's Communication Handbook* (3e). Radcliffe Medical Press, Oxford.

Analysis of patient contacts

By this, I mean analysis of the records we keep following consultations with patients. These are rarely a full record of what went on in the consultation, but they can be examined to determine what we did, as well as what we didn't do and why. One approach, described in Chapter 6, on PUNs & DENs, is to look *contemporaneously* at our consultations. After each one, we briefly note whether the patient had an area of need of which we were aware but did not address. We can then use this insight to decide whether such unmet needs might be due to an educational deficiency on our part.

Another method is to look *retrospectively* at our records using the benefit of hindsight. We may be prompted to do this by a significant event. Suppose, for example, that a young adult is admitted to hospital and found to have ulcerative colitis. Following this we may decide to revise our knowledge of the presentation of the condition and conduct a retrospective case review looking at the patient's notes and asking ourselves if there were any symptoms, signs or investigations that could have alerted us earlier to the diagnosis.

Sometimes there are guidelines or protocols which define good practice, such as those for the secondary prevention of coronary heart disease (CHD). Using these to audit our care, we can look back at our contacts with patients with CHD to determine how aware we are of the recommendations, and to what degree they are being implemented.

Prescribing and practice activity (PACT) data

PACT data is routinely available and is a useful educational resource. It can be used in several ways: to look at the pattern of our prescribing as individuals, to compare our prescribing with that of our partners and to compare practices with each other. An example of learning through comparison with our colleagues might be in relation to a particular therapeutic area. For instance, we might question why our prescribing of HRT is only half that of another partner and discover that either the answer is obvious (the partner is female and the peri–menopausal women in the practice choose to consult her), or else that it requires further thought. Such reflection might reveal that we choose not to recommend HRT because of our concerns over the risk of breast cancer and this may lead to re-education with the result that our fears might be allayed and our prescribing habit changed.

Many doctors begin their therapeutic analysis by looking at areas of high prescribing (particularly cost), inappropriate prescribing (e.g. long-term benzo-diazepines) or areas of therapeutic advance (e.g. *H. pylori* eradication). There are several sources of guidance regarding best practice, with the *Drug & Therapeutics Bulletin*, *Prescribers Journal* and *BNF* guidelines being particularly authoritative. The community pharmacist is often keen to help and can encourage GPs to discuss their prescribing together without them becoming too defensive with each other.

Looking at *practice activity data* means analysing the pattern of our tests and investigations along with the referrals that we make to other team members and beyond the practice. Through this, we can make comparisons of numbers and discuss why differences exist. If we find that our referral rate to the dermatology department is twice that of our partners this might be because our skill in dermatology has made us more astute and vigilant practitioners, identifying lesions at an early stage and appropriately referring them on. On the other hand, if we look at our skin referrals and find that the cases comprise a disproportionately high number of non-suspicious skin lesions which are being referred for excision, we might question whether this is appropriate. We might then decide that such lesions could be removed in a minor surgery clinic within the practice and make plans to train ourselves for this purpose.

As well as looking at numbers, or the quantity of our work, we can also look at its quality. For example in attempting to determine the degree to which patients with angina should be investigated and treated before referral to secondary care, discussion with GPs and hospital doctors might clarify the standards which could then be investigated by an audit of our referral letters. This might lead to re-education and an improvement in care.

Objective tests

Because we direct our education to the problems we commonly encounter, we may notice that our knowledge is developing in some areas but may not be aware that it is diminishing in others. It is said that our confidence in dealing with problems diminishes rather more slowly than our competence and many doctors recognise this to be true. To maintain competence as generalists we require an all-round knowledge of our subject, so how can we determine the areas in which our knowledge is lacking? Objective tests provide a mechanism for doing this and nowadays are tailored to practising GPs rather than just those taking exams, with their focus being on what we *need* to know rather than what we *could* know. Some provide mini-tutorials as well as assessments and one of the best is *PEP-CD*: a CD containing a phased evaluation programme covering several areas of clinical, therapeutic and practice management (available from RCGP, PEP Office, 12 Queen Street, Edinburgh EH2 1JE).

Educational meetings

It is preferable to attend meetings not merely out of interest, but because we think that we might learn something. During the meeting, we should be on the lookout for those times when we feel uneasy with the subject material as these points might signify the presence of competence gaps which need addressing. Because meetings are quickly forgotten, it is best to make a note of these gaps as soon after the meeting as possible.

The meeting should have some learning objectives specified by the organiser, and at the end of the meeting we should decide to what extent these objectives have been met. If they were *not* met, consideration should be given as to whether the fault lay with the presenter or with ourselves.

Audit work and research activity

Audit is a powerful way of identifying gaps and of checking that those gaps have subsequently been closed. Because it is a method of measuring our performance against certain standards, audit can not only identify gaps but can indicate how large those gaps are. The mechanism and potential of clinical audit are discussed in Chapter 8.

Research provides the evidence-base for our work and in order to be generalisable to primary care, it is increasingly being performed within the community. GPs can learn much by engaging in this research, either by providing data for research projects or by conducting research of their own.

Reading

Medical texts, journals and, more recently, Internet sources provide the basis for keeping up to date. The problem lies with prioritising the vast array of information which is available to us and there is a need to triage the literature in order to decide first what to read and second whether to act on it. To learn how to prioritise journals and articles, it is worth reading the article by MaCauley (1994) *Br J Gen Pract* **44:** 83–5 in which the READER acronym is described. This system ascribes scores to articles on the basis of their:

- Relevance to general practice
- Educational value in bringing about a change in behaviour
- Applicability to our own practice
- Discrimination in terms of methodology.

We can't change our practice in the light of *all* new developments, so deciding what we should take notice of enables us to make our learning effective.

The arts

For many GPs, medicine is more an art than a science and all aspects of the human condition have the capacity to inform our practice. By learning from the creativity of others and from our own creative efforts, we can gain insights that help us as people and as doctors.

The practical benefit for patient care comes from a deeper understanding of how people experience physical and psychological illness, and this can lead to improved abilities in communicating with patients and managing illness. Using experiences from the world outside medicine as part of our development plans is legitimate if we can demonstrate that we can learn from them in ways which improve our work.

Prioritising our learning needs

Using the range of methods discussed, we may gain many experiences from which our educational needs can be identified. Once these needs have been recognised, we need to prioritise *which* of them we propose attending to and *in what order*. Our decision will be influenced by personal needs, the needs of the practice and the needs of external agencies, as depicted in Figure 2.2.

Because the priorities which are set are influenced by other agencies, it is better if we can decide on them in consultation with our colleagues. Although there are no rules with regard to deciding which educational needs should get priority, the following represents a practical approach.

Safety first

Potentially, there is a tension between the desires of the individual and the wishes of others with regard to which needs are prioritised, because individuals will want to retain ownership of their educational activity. However, most parties would agree that safety and basic competence are the first priority.

Therefore when we look at our educational needs, we have to ask: 'What are the implications for patient care of *not* prioritising this need?', and the more serious the consequences for the patient, the more urgently should the need be addressed. Hence, if we were in charge of an immunisation clinic and did not know how we

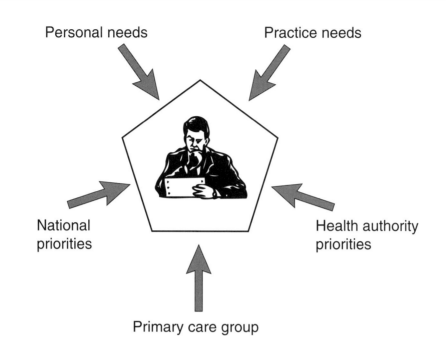

Figure 2.2 Prioritising our needs: the influences on GPs.

would resuscitate a child who had suffered an anaphylactic reaction, we should attend to this need before learning more about meningitis immunisation, for example.

Moving on, if we are satisfied that negligence is not an issue, we need to consider whether any of our educational deficiencies represent a threat to basic medical competence. For instance, not knowing how to manage a UTI in a child may not result in sudden death but could compromise the health of the child in the longer term.

Obeying orders

Increasingly, there are directives from other bodies that have to be carried through at practice level. Guidelines from organisations such as the National Institute for Clinical Excellence (NICE) will recommend how certain conditions should be managed across the nation, and other programmes and targets will be set at local level with involvement from GP practices. We need to ensure that we have the skills to carry these programmes through and if we have educational needs that fall within the topic areas, then these should be given priority.

Addressing these needs should not be problematic, as one of the responsibilities of clinical governance is to ensure that educational programmes to support the initiatives are in place. As well as providing education on clinical areas such as the management of angina, the programmes will provide an opportunity for GPs and others in the team to share ideas with colleagues from neighbouring practices.

Practice development

Once the wider expectations are met, we are free to attend to the other needs of our practices. The practice development plan (or business plan) will set goals that require particular skills from the team members and we may therefore decide to tailor part of our educational programme to meet these requirements. For example, if medical services as well as income generation are being compromised because we are not qualified for minor surgery or child health promotion, then undertaking the appropriate training may become our priority.

Sometimes practice development is driven by special needs within the community. For instance, it may be that the minority Asian population on the practice list is being neglected because no-one has taken an interest in transcultural medicine. Individuals may not have recognised this as a personal educational need, but once it has been identified by the practice it may become important that someone (perhaps everyone) places it on their educational agenda.

In future, the practice professional development plan developed by the team will identify and prioritise certain learning needs. The mechanism by which this might occur is described in Chapter 1.

Personal agenda

Although seemingly at the bottom of the list, most of the priorities we set from our list of educational needs will arise from our personal agenda, but how we choose the priorities requires consideration. A good place to start is to think about those deficiencies which cause us the greatest unease. These quite often arise from significant events, and correcting these deficiencies helps us not only in educational terms but also in being able to put the event behind us and move on.

It is also useful to think of any longer-term plans that we have for our professional development as these goals might dictate the skills that we need to acquire. For example, we may have ambitions with regard to GP training and may therefore wish to go on a course for potential trainers, or we may hope to become a company doctor and hence have the need to learn more about occupational health medicine.

Our personal needs may relate to our everyday work. For example, the higher levels of computer literacy which are becoming mandatory for GPs may encourage us to develop our skills in this area. Finally, there may be needs which address deficiencies but don't bring any immediate practical benefits. For instance, if we learn more about medical ethics we may become wiser doctors but may not be able to demonstrate the benefits of that wisdom, although as we know, much that is of benefit in life remains intangible.

Summary

The experiences from which GPs can learn are all around us and are part of the fabric of our working lives. In this chapter we have looked at the sources of these experiences, some of which will be familiar but others of which may offer new routes for learning. Three of these sources, namely PUNs & DENs, significant event analysis and clinical audit are particularly fruitful and will be considered in detail in Chapters 6–8.

Identifying and prioritising our educational needs ensures that the limited time we have to attend to these needs is optimally spent, and in the next chapter we will discuss how we can take an educational need and address it through the use of a personal development plan.

3 Personal development plans (PDPs)

Key points

- Those who use them wouldn't go back.
- PDPs will be a key feature of Revalidation.
- GPs are in charge of setting their personal educational agenda.
- Individuals can decide what they wish to learn and how they wish to learn it.
- Development plans are not set in stone – they evolve through the year.
- Colleagues can use each other for support and as resources.
- Learning is most useful when it is applied.
- Evaluating what we do increases the usefulness of the exercise.
- PDPs are simple: they are drawn from what we do and feed back directly to our work.

Introduction

Nothing could have been more straightforward than PGEA – go to meetings, sit through a lecture, collect an accreditation form, avoid or succumb to the bribe of a ballpoint pen (depending on your state of political correctness) and away. Despite this, GPs voiced the reservations that they had to give up their valuable time and often failed to learn anything useful.

For a few years, a new path for postgraduate education has been available in some regions – the personal development plan (PDP). Those who have chosen this route have almost universally found it to be a more interesting and relevant way of continuing their learning. Even the small amount of writing involved has not been off-putting and, indeed, has been found to be useful.

In the following three chapters we will look at the principles underpinning the PDP, how to make a start on writing one and how a completed plan could be formatively assessed. The fact that all GPs are now encouraged to have such plans should not be alarming and in this chapter I will try to explain their usefulness, how we can produce them and how, despite initially appearing complicated, they are really quite straightforward.

This chapter presents a comprehensive overview of the PDP and is designed for you to read and refer back to. If you are writing your PDP for the first time, it is recommended that you read this chapter and then follow the guidance in Chapter 4.

Why do we need PDPs?

The General Medical Council states that in order to be fit to practise, doctors have a professional duty to make sure that their knowledge and skills are kept up to date. GPs will in future be required to *demonstrate* this fitness through the process of Revalidation.

To comply with this GPs will not have to take exams, thank goodness, but instead demonstrate over a five-yearly cycle that they have engaged in systematic learning. This demonstration (or proof) will be in the form of a *record of personal learning* which, if thought adequate, will allow doctors to continue in practice. As shown opposite, the PDP forms an integral part of this record.

The record of learning is likely to be in three parts:

- A *personal development plan*, which is written at the start of each year. In it are stated the educational priorities for the year, how we wish to meet them and how we intend to evaluate what we have done. The plan is flexible so as to allow for additional priorities to be added during the year, or previously stated priorities to be removed if no longer appropriate.

- A *record of activities*, which is a log of the things we have done in order to meet the educational objectives. The log records these activities (what we have read, the meetings we have been to, etc.), what we have learned from them, and how we have applied the new knowledge or skills that have been gained.

- An *educational portfolio*, which is a compilation of documents or other material which we collect in order to demonstrate that we have undertaken our PDP. This might include our development plan and record of activities along with other documents such as completed audits or protocols. Note that the PDP and its associated portfolio of evidence is not a complete record of all that we spend time learning. Such a task would be impossible to achieve and de-motivating to attempt. Instead, it is an opportunity to plan our learning in a proactive way rather than just to learn as a reaction to the demands of practice life.

As well as being required for Revalidation, PDPs offer the following advantages:

- They are based on learning cycles of which we have ownership.

- They require us to establish what we *need* to learn rather than just what we want to learn, thus making it more likely that we will *improve* our skills rather than just reinforce those which are already adequate.

- They ask us to state *what we hope to achieve* as a result of the time spent learning. This strongly encourages us to make sure that our plans will produce some practical benefits for ourselves and our practices. This is a move away from learning for learning's sake, which although of value has a lower priority in this context.

- They make us crystallise our educational aims into *specific objectives*, which is useful in two ways. First, being clear about what we need to learn helps us to identify the best educational method by which to achieve it, and second, it stops us from wasting time through going off at a tangent.

- As a final step, PDPs require us to *evaluate our learning cycle.* Being critical about what we have achieved and how we have achieved it helps us to learn more effectively in the future.

What does a PDP look like?

A PDP is a list of a few educational priorities for each of which we answer a number of questions, as shown in the examples which follow. Each of these examples represents an educational need which has been prioritised for action, and the answers to the questions demonstrate how that need will be addressed. The examples are drawn from different sources such as self-awareness, feedback and reading, and are of different types ranging from the biomedical and service-orientated to the reflective and personal.

The number of questions asked may appear daunting, but they follow a logical sequence and allow almost any experience to be translated into a development plan. Each example uses a pro-forma, a copy of which appears at the end of the chapter for your use. After the examples, each question from the pro-forma is considered in further detail to make clear both its purpose and how it should be answered. In practice, you should find the questions simple to answer and the forms easy to use.

A PDP may look like a collection of the following forms, perhaps compiled into a table, but as there is no national form you may not be required to answer all these questions in your region, although to get the most from your development plan it is worth thinking about them all.

Writing our development plan

We will now look at these questions more closely – questions which begin broadly and then get us to focus down.

What is the general area in which I need to learn?

This question gets us to confirm that we are in the right ballpark. In association with the following question, it also prompts us to double-check that the area chosen is a priority learning need (however that priority has been defined)

Personal development plan: educational priority

What is the general area in which I need to learn?
Hypertension

How have I established this need?
Awareness that hypertension guidelines have been published by the British
Hypertension Society (BHS) in 1999

What is the aim of my learning?
To control hypertension in line with the guideline recommendations

What are the specific objectives that I wish to achieve?
1 Know the target level for BP control
2 Write a protocol for diagnosis and investigation of hypertension
3 Prescribe in accordance with the BHS guidelines
4 Amend the practice formulary for antihypertensive medication

How do I intend to achieve these objectives?
1 Read the BHS guidelines
2 Attend the GP therapeutics forum meeting
3 Organise a multidisciplinary practice meeting
4 Work with colleagues on the new protocol and updated formulary

How will I evaluate my development plan?
Audit the BP control of our hypertensive patients

How will I demonstrate that I have undertaken this plan?
1 Keep a copy of the BHS guidelines
2 Make a note of points of interest raised in the therapeutics forum
3 Present documentation such as action points from the practice meeting
4 Keep a copy of the diagnosis/investigation protocol and the new formulary
5 Show the results of BP audit

What is my timescale?
1 Three months to establish new protocol
2 Conduct audit 12 months after new protocol is implemented to allow for
  treatment changes and the fact that many patients are going to be on multiple
  therapy

Personal development plan: educational priority

What is the general area in which I need to learn?
Rheumatoid arthritis (RA)

How have I established this need?
Feedback from rheumatologist who suggested that I should administer gold
injections

What is the aim of my learning?
To be able to give gold injections to suitable rheumatoid patients

What are the specific objectives that I wish to achieve?
1 Know the indications for using gold in RA
2 Write a shared-care protocol for gold injections
3 Teach the practice nurse how to administer the injection and monitor treatment

How do I intend to achieve these objectives?
1 Revise the literature
2 Liaise with the rheumatologist to establish a shared-care protocol
3 Arrange a teaching session with the practice nurse

How will I evaluate my development plan?
After implementing shared care, conduct a survey of the rheumatoid patients
receiving gold injections to establish whether these are being given in the hospital
or in the practice

How will I demonstrate that I have undertaken this plan?
1 Keep any notes from my reading and liaison with the rheumatologist
2 Keep a copy of the shared-care protocol
3 Show the results of the survey

What is my timescale?
Three months: no immediate rush because the rheumatologist is providing the
service and we need time to inform our rheumatoid patients, for whom gold
injections are needed, of the transfer of care

Personal development plan: educational priority

What is the general area in which I need to learn?
Anticoagulation

How have I established this need?
Many more patients require warfarin because of AF. Most attend the hospital clinic for monitoring but say that they would prefer to come to us

What is the aim of my learning?
To be able to dose patients whose INR is already stabilised

What are the specific objectives that I wish to achieve?
1 Define the population for whom anticoagulation is appropriate
2 Obtain any equipment/software required
3 Write a protocol for the practice anticoagulation clinic covering call and recall, dosing and communication with the patient

How do I intend to achieve these objectives?
1 Collect data on patients attending the hospital clinic
2 Talk to the consultant haematologist and meet with GPs in the neighbouring practice who offer this service
3 Arrange to perform initial dosing under supervision
4 Investigate computer program to assist in dosing and monitoring
5 Arrange a meeting with the healthcare team to discuss a new clinic protocol

How will I evaluate my development plan?
Audit the numbers of patients being dosed at the hospital and in the practice before and after implementing the proposed changes

How will I demonstrate that I have undertaken this plan?
1 Keep any documentation from the data collection
2 Keep a copy of the anticoagulation audit
3 Show the new anticoagulation clinic protocol
4 Consider conducting a patient satisfaction survey

What is my timescale?
Six months – setting up a new clinic always takes longer than you think!

Personal development plan: educational priority

What is the general area in which I need to learn?
Consulting skills

How have I established this need?
Increasingly I'm finding that I get irritated by my patients in consultation and I wondered whether the way I consult might be part of the problem

What is the aim of my learning?
To be able to analyse my consultations

What are the specific objectives that I wish to achieve?
1 Know what is meant by 'consultation tasks'
2 Obtain feedback on my consulting skills
3 Demonstrate evidence of improvement in these skills

How do I intend to achieve these objectives?
1 Read about consultation tasks
2 Record a video of my consultations
3 Ask my partner (a trainer) to analyse it with me using a consultation task checklist
4 Following the feedback make some changes to the way I consult
5 Record another series of consultations and obtain further feedback

How will I evaluate my development plan?
Keep the checklists from the feedback sessions I have with my colleague – do they indicate that any improvement has occurred?

How will I demonstrate that I have undertaken this plan?
1 Keep any notes from the literature on consulting skills which I read
2 Note the dates of video consultations (the video may not be available for viewing because of patient confidentiality)
3 Keep the feedback notes

What is my timescale?
Four months – I want to give myself time to practise my new skills

How have I established this need?

As our learning plan is going to require a commitment from us, it is vital that we check, as we would in our practice lives, that this commitment is based on a firm foundation. This question asks us to test that foundation by looking at two areas:

- Who said that I need to do this?
- What is the strength of the evidence that I need to do it?

We must feel happy that we have ownership of our plan, i.e. that the priority set is our own and not purely the will of others, and satisfy ourselves that it is based on evidence of a deficiency which *we* regard as being important to correct. Some types of evidence are stronger than others, as for example the results of a clinical audit on asthma admissions, which might clarify an educational need in a way that a vague sense of unease at managing asthma emergencies might not.

The question also gives an insight into the sources of experience from which we draw, which can encourage us to both cultivate these further and to consider why other sources are less fruitful.

What is the aim of my learning?

As part of a wider consideration this question asks us to say what we hope to achieve as a result of completing our learning plan. We should answer this by asking ourselves 'Once I have completed this exercise, what will I be able to do that I could not do before?'

The aim may be in the form of:

- A *new skill* such as injecting joints.
- Providing a *new service* such as running an anticoagulation clinic.
- Some new level of *knowledge or understanding*, e.g. appreciating the cultural perspective of an ethnic minority population.
- A different *attitude* such as increased confidence in managing drug addicts.

What are the specific objectives that I wish to achieve?

Aims and objectives sometimes get confused with each other, but an aim is the ultimate purpose of our activity and the objectives are those tasks which need to be completed in order to achieve that aim. For example, if our aim was to take a holiday in Peru, our objectives would include specific tasks such as buying the airline tickets, obtaining foreign currency and having our holiday vaccinations.

With the PDP our aim is usually written as an educational need, and it may be large and relatively unfocused. Writing clear objectives allows us to plan how we will meet our aim. In this way, we can convert a nebulous goal into a series of manageable steps that between them will ensure that we succeed in achieving what we set out to do. Very often, when plans fail they do so because the objectives have been poorly thought out and as a result are found difficult to achieve or not relevant to the original aim. To illustrate this, look at Table 3.1:

Table 3.1: Personal development plan

Educational need	Learning objectives
To learn how to control hypertension in line with guidelines on best practice	1 Have a look at the recent literature 2 Talk to colleagues at the hypertension clinic 3 Rewrite the practice protocol

If we were to carry through these learning objectives, could we be sure of meeting our aim? To help decide upon our objectives, it is useful to ask:

- 'What do I want to be able to do that I can't do now?' and
- 'How will I know when I've got there?'

One way of thinking about how to *phrase* our objective is to complete the sentence:

'At the end of this process I will . . .'

In doing so, the second half of the sentence will often contain a verb like 'write' (for example, a guideline), 'record', 'summarise' and so on. This phrase will usually provide a form of words that we can use in our plan.

Objectives define the staging posts in meeting the aim, and good objectives are said to be **SMART**, meaning that they are:

- Specific: clear and concise.
- Measurable: written as verbs (e.g. analyse, design, prescribe, inject etc.) rather

than as 'woolly' objectives (e.g. become aware of, understand, appreciate, etc.) which cannot be easily defined or measured.

- Achievable: by ensuring that resources (e.g. expertise, time and funding) are available and that the goals are attainable.
- Relevant to the aim.
- Time-bound: with the date for completion being both explicit and realistic.

Now look at Table 3.2 which is taken from the previous example of a PDP:

Table 3.2: Personal development plan

Educational need	Learning objectives
To learn how to control hypertension in line with guidelines on best practice	1 Know the target level for BP control 2 Understand the prescribing implications of the BHS guidelines 3 Know how my current standards of BP control compare to the BHS guidelines

Try comparing these objectives with those offered in Table 3.1. If you were to implement these objectives, you would be better placed to meet your need than in the original example and this is because the objectives are SMARTer. Can you identify in what ways?

It is worth noting that objectives are not always large and can sometimes be deceptive. The first objective in Table 3.2 does not seem ambitious but it is certainly important. However, in meeting it we would find that the target level is not straightforward but depends on several factors such as diabetic status and whether we are thinking about a treatment or an audit standard.

How do I intend to achieve the objectives?

We have seen the importance of writing SMART objectives and the way in which they can help us to plan appropriate learning activities. These activities are otherwise known as learning methods and in the next section of the learning plan we try to specify which methods we intend to use.

At the time the plan is written, the exact activities to be used may not be clear and they will almost certainly change as learning proceeds. The main reason for thinking about our methods at this early stage is that it helps us to identify a starting point for implementing our plan. Our learning may then take a different course, influenced as it is by the availability of resources such as appropriate tutors, courses, the recommendations of colleagues and our preferred learning styles.

There is no right or wrong way to learn and the important point is to choose a method of learning that suits our purpose as defined by our objectives. For transferring information and getting a quick 'update', we may prefer solitary methods of learning, e.g. didactic teaching such as reading a book or attending a postgraduate lecture. On the other hand, for putting information into the context of our practice as with learning how to alter our case management in the light of new guidelines, it may be better to choose an interactive method such as group learning. Much of our education is enhanced if it is interactive and learning with our colleagues allows us to gain insights that may not have occurred to us, as well as helping us to apply our learning more effectively. Our chosen companions for learning may be other doctors, but emphasis is given nowadays to the importance of multidisciplinary learning, i.e. learning facilitated by and shared between members of the team.

The learning method also needs to be appropriate to the attribute we hope to gain. Hence knowledge can be acquired from a book but if we were trying to gain a skill such as being able to insert a contraceptive implant, we would do better to gain practical experience with a tutor rather than study the manufacturer's leaflet.

Some examples of methods that we could use are shown in Box 3.1.

In choosing the methods, we will bear in mind our previous experiences and may tend to favour those approaches that worked for us in the past. This might be because we enjoyed that way of learning, because it was feasible or simply because it worked.

Learning methods that have proved their effectiveness by leading to change deserve to be prioritised in this way. However, we will not know all the possible methods and the pros and cons of each approach, and for this reason it can be helpful to supplement our experience with the advice of colleagues when deciding which educational methods would be most appropriate. Between them, colleagues will have a wider range of learning styles and therefore of favoured methods, and will know which courses, speakers, etc. are worth using and which should be avoided. In addition to providing advice, quite often our colleagues also turn out to be the best tutors, and it is remarkable how even a small group of GPs can attend to many of each other's educational needs.

Box 3.1 Learning methods

Reading	for ourselves or as part of a journal club using books, journals and literature searches
Lectures	the better ones having a primary care focus with an opportunity for discussion
Meetings and discussions	with partners, colleagues (e.g. principals, groups, consultants, clinical advisers, tutors, mentors, etc.), members of the healthcare team and the wider public
Workshops	small-group, task-orientated work
Courses	including distance learning by post or electronically via the Internet
Personal tuition	perhaps being taught a practical skill by a colleague
Work experience	e.g. clinical assistantships, short-term individual attachments in secondary or primary care
Audit	either conducted by ourselves or by learning lessons from audit conducted by others
Research	usually with support, often as part of a research group
Computer-based methods	e.g. Internet searching using search engines such as Medline, being part of an e-mail discussion group, using interactive packages on the Internet or CD-ROM

How will I evaluate my development plan?

Once the plan is complete, it is considered important to evaluate the outcomes of learning and the process of learning itself, the purpose being to help to make our future learning more effective. The GP tutor can provide guidance, but the technique is one of self-evaluation using questions such as the following.

How did we identify our learning needs for this PDP, and what other methods might we include in our next PDP?

Many doctors determine their needs intuitively and therefore may not recognise that assessing learning needs is a skill that can be learned. A range of techniques, both subjective (e.g. reflection, feedback and questionnaires) and objective (e.g. analysis of PACT and referral data) is available for use and each of them can give a different perspective on our performance. Thinking about ways in which we identify our needs helps us to identify the techniques that we use, and can help to broaden the range of techniques that we employ.

Which objectives were easiest/most difficult to achieve and why?

The importance of writing SMART objectives has been stressed, but it is not intuitive and therefore can be difficult to learn. Reflecting upon those objectives that worked, or did not work well, is a good way of learning to recognise the link between successful outcomes of learning and the use of SMART objectives.

If our objectives were not achieved, we could speculate on the reasons for this and on how we might achieve success in the future. It might have been that the objectives we set were unrealistic, resources were not available or commitment was lacking.

Which were the most/least valuable learning activities and why?

As experienced learners, we have our preferred learning methods that reflect our educational needs as well as our personalities. Although educationalists sometimes assume that certain methods (e.g. talk and chalk) are bad and others (e.g. small group work) are good, this is debatable and the important factor is not the method itself but whether we consider that our time was profitably spent in terms of helping to achieve our objectives.

GP tutors may suggest other routes to learning. For instance, because the perspectives and feedback of others can be so illuminating some interactive methods could be suggested to doctors who seem to learn mainly in isolation.

Broadening the range of methods used can be useful, but it may be equally appropriate to continue with a learning method (e.g. distance learning) that we have found works for us.

In what ways have we been able to apply our learning to practice?

The ultimate aim of the PDP process is to learn *and* to be able to apply that learning to practice, preferably in a way that produces benefits for patients.

If improvements occurred, it is helpful to put them into context by showing how they are an advance on previous practice, and if learning was not applied it is just as important to discuss why this was either not appropriate or not possible.

Are there any learning needs that we wish to carry forward to the next PDP?

On reflection, we may wish to carry some existing needs forward, perhaps with new objectives, or to address new areas of need uncovered whilst undertaking the PDP. Each PDP should inform future plans by helping to make the process of learning more effective, but should not automatically dictate the content of these plans. Therefore, we should not feel obliged to take educational needs forward from one year's plan to the next.

Do we have any useful feedback on the PDP process?

The process of engaging doctors and supporting them with their PDPs is new and requires evaluation if it is to remain useful and credible. Rather than assume that no news is good news, tutors prefer feedback as this helps to keep the focus on the needs of the learner.

Self-evaluation is conducted by answering the questions posed, perhaps using a proforma such as that shown at the end of this chapter. To gain the maximum value these evaluations can be usefully discussed in a group, as there may be lessons that have a wider application. For instance, a positive outcome of learning due to the use of a good resource deserves to be more widely known. On the other hand, if barriers are identified such as a lack of support or funding, these could be addressed and overcome, especially if the group discussing their PDPs were members of the same practice.

Evaluation can be seen to serve as a springboard to future learning, and it may be that in time to come such a meeting could encompass both evaluation of the previous year's PDP and consideration of next year's initial learning plan.

How will I demonstrate that I have undertaken this development plan?

Being asked for 'proof' can seem threatening and there is a need to achieve a balance between keeping an educational focus for the PDP and using it as a means to demonstrate accountability to such people as appraisers and revalidators. Here are some guidelines that can help.

What should the evidence demonstrate?

Evidence comes in different grades and in the most basic form it may be little more than proof that the learner has engaged in the learning process. For example, if time is being claimed for PGEA purposes, we may need to produce evidence such as a record of the hours spent in completing our objectives.

An improvement on this would be evidence arising from reflection on educational activities as described below. In its most advanced form, evidence refers to the application of learning as might be demonstrated through a change in practice. This goal is certainly important, but may not always be within the power of the learner to deliver, perhaps because it requires the efforts of others to achieve, requires additional resources or cannot easily be measured. For instance, improving diabetic outcomes needs co-operative patients as well as good medicine, and although learning about the needs of ethnic minorities may make us more understanding as doctors, this could be difficult to prove.

The one caveat is that for Revalidation, proof of application of learning to practice in a way that benefits patients, *is* likely to be required over a five-year cycle, and therefore we need to ensure that at some point in this period we could fulfil this.

What types of evidence could I keep?

The most useful evidence is that which helps us to get the most from our educational activity as well as serving the needs of accountability. This means that, wherever possible, our evidence should arise from our mainstream activity rather than be produced solely for assessors.

For example, in seeking to improve the management of osteoporosis we may decide to write a practice guideline or a patient information leaflet. Either of these would form good evidence of learning and other such examples include audit work or the production of administrative protocols. For those doctors that spend time presenting ideas or educating others, the material that is produced such as handouts, overhead projector slides or meeting notes could be used as evidence.

What if there is no obvious outcome of learning?

Sometimes evidence does not arise quite so naturally from learning, and in these circumstances we can produce evidence that shows our thoughts about what we have learned. This is sometimes called 'proof of reflection' as distinct from 'proof of action'. We often learn through reading, and it is in no one's interest to keep the primary material that we have read – we would soon run out of filing cabinets in any case! Instead, we could highlight the important points in the text, keep a record of the main references read with bullet points of the material thought relevant, or write a few lines on how the new information might influence our future practice.

Where learning has occurred through attending a lecture or course, going to a meeting, etc., evidence of reflection might be an evaluation in terms of what was learned or how our practice might be influenced by the event. This could be written on a learning log as demonstrated overleaf. Certificates of attendance are not adequate in themselves, as they are merely proof of attendance not proof of learning, and it would be better to complete a proforma such as the blank learning log included at the end of this chapter.

We are often in a better position to assess the importance of a meeting after letting it sink in. It may therefore be more meaningful if we answer these questions the following day rather than immediately after the session, when we are in a rush to get home. As a means of raising our awareness, reflection is a very powerful tool and formalising it in this way can help us to capture the lessons learned in a way that 'just thinking about it' cannot.

What is my timescale?

When we write the educational priorities for our PDPs, it is usually intended that the tasks we set be completed within the following 12 months. Bearing this in mind, we need to be realistic about the timescale for each aim that we define. Giving ourselves too little time runs the risk of leaving us exhausted and demotivated; giving ourselves too much may deprive us of any sense of urgency and the task may never be completed.

We need to consider that although we will be working towards several educational objectives simultaneously, we may need to complete some ahead of others. For example, we may consider it to be more important to revise our diabetic clinic protocol before learning about cognitive behaviour therapy!

Finally, we have to build in some flexibility so that we can deal with pressing educational needs as they arise. These may arise from personal experiences, such as learning how to manage a Bengali mum who while breast-feeding her third child has been diagnosed with pulmonary TB. Alternatively, they may come from

Learning log

Date	Activity	Subject area	Learning aim	What did I learn?	How could I apply what I have learned in practice?
2/3/00	Practitioner group meeting	Type 2 diabetes	To review management guidelines	Recent literature (UKPDS) demonstrates the need for tight control of blood sugar *and* BP	1 Audit BP and HbA1 measured in our diabetic clinic 2 Set new standards for diabetic management (more aggressive BP treatment and more referrals for insulin therapy) 3 Complete audit cycle
7/4/00	Significant event analysis: missed diagnosis	Polymyalgia rheumatica	To review clinical presentation and ensure early diagnosis	Polymyalgia can present with malaise alone	Increase my index of suspicion so that when this symptom persists, I request an ESR
10/6/00	Reading *BMJ* article of 22/05/00	Prevention of corticosteroid-induced osteoporosis	Raise awareness of risk	1 Patients on long-term prednisolone 7.5 mg/day or more need advice on vitamin D and calcium 2 Those on 15 mg/day or more, or with risk factors, need bisphosphonates	1 Identify patients on long-term steroids (mainly for COPD, RA and polymyalgia) 2 Flag records of those at risk 3 Discuss article with local osteoporosis expert and colleagues 4 Implement recommendations

external influences such as planning a smoking cessation strategy for the practice in response to a government directive.

The process of producing a PDP

There is no standard method for producing the PDP, and different regions have their own approach, which your GP tutor can advise you of. GPs can either formulate their plans individually or with a group of colleagues from within or without their practices, facilitated by the GP tutor or by others who have undertaken PDPs before. Doctors from the same practice may understand each other's educational needs better, and may be more successful at tailoring their development plans to the needs of the practice.

On the other hand, doctors from different practices may find it easier to be more open with each other about their educational deficiencies, and may be able to offer each other a wider range of resources with which to address those needs.

As previously mentioned, the plan is flexible to allow for educational priorities to be changed as circumstances dictate during the year. If not forewarned, when undertaking a development plan for the first time, it can be quite disconcerting to find that by the end of the year the PDP may bear little resemblance to the original draft! This should not be regarded as a failure but as a sign of success in allowing education to be adaptable, and the GP tutor can help to advise about both the content and the evolution of the plan.

How do PDPs tie in with learning cycles?

As we saw in Chapter 1, our experiences lead us to reflect, determine and address our educational needs and finally to apply what we have learned. This is the learning cycle.

These steps are the same as those in our PDPs with the only additional requirements being that we *evaluate* what we have done and provide *evidence* that we have undertaken a learning process.

Let us modify the original Figure 1.1 to illustrate this point (Figure 3.1).

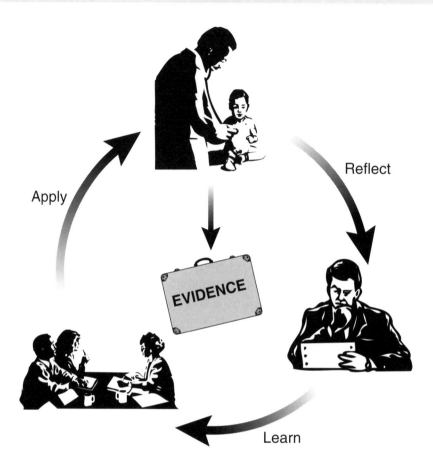

Figure 3.1

The doctor in this example used his sense of unease to define his educational need, which was to be able to tell the difference between an innocent and a pathological cardiac murmur in a small child. This experience was the start of his learning cycle, but it could also have been the start of his PDP had he chosen to write down how he was going to address his need, apply his new knowledge and evaluate how worthwhile the exercise had been. To complete his record of learning he could have collected any of the following 'evidence' for his portfolio:

• An account of the significant event (feeling uneasy at hearing a murmur which he could not interpret) which he could record in his learning log.

- Notes from the meeting he attended on paediatric assessment.
- A case review of the next child in whom he detected a murmur.

Thus we can see that if we wish them to, development plans can flow directly from learning cycles.

Summary

The PDP is no more nor less than a mechanism for establishing the way in which our educational priorities can be met and the success of our plans evaluated. The examples given have shown that the process is straightforward, and although the details relate to GPs, the principles involved are applicable to all members of the healthcare team. We have seen how everyday experiences can be used to initiate our learning cycles, PDPs and educational portfolios. Thus our learning can become an integral part of our practice lives, using experiences drawn from our work and applying the results of that learning back to that work in a cycle which should have benefits for practitioners and patients alike.

Later in the book, we will examine three powerful methods by which our learning needs can be determined and the principles discussed will again be seen to be relevant to other members of the team.

Further information

Chief Medical Officer (1998) *A Review of Continuing Professional Development in General Practice.* Department of Health, London.

An influential document that sets the scene for the future of personal and practice development plans. It can also be accessed at the web-site: www.doh. gov.uk/cmo/cmodev.htm

Personal development plans have been in use in Sheffield for some years, and the following web-site, which gives further details on PDPs, has been developed partly from this experience: www.wisdom.org.uk

Personal development plan: educational priority

What is the general area in which I need to learn?

How have I established this need?

What is the aim of my learning?

What are the specific objectives that I wish to achieve?

How do I intend to achieve these objectives?

How will I evaluate my development plan?

How will I demonstrate that I have undertaken this plan?

What is my timescale?

Learning log

Date	Activity	Subject area	Learning aim	What did I learn?	How could I apply what I have learned in practice?

Development plan: evaluation

How did you identify your learning needs for this PDP, and what other methods might you include in your next PDP?

Which objectives were easiest to achieve and why?

Which objectives were most difficult to achieve and why?

Which were the most valuable learning activities and why?

Which were the least valuable learning activities and why?

In what ways have you been able to apply your learning in practice?

What benefits to your patients do you feel have occurred as a result of your learning?

Are there any learning needs that you wish to carry forward to your next PDP?

Do you have any suggestions or comments about the administration of your PDP or the support that you have received?

4 Making a start

Key points

- We must learn to walk before attempting to run. A basic PDP is easy to write – anyone can do it.
- We need to keep our learning aims simple. The most important thing is to make a start.
- It is better to undertake a PDP as part of a group than to go it alone.
- You will not be unsupported – facilitators such as GP tutors can guide you.
- The standards required will be within your reach.
- PDPs are liberating. Even reading this book could count as part of your development plan.

Introduction

Having read the previous chapter, you may feel a little overwhelmed! If so, don't worry, it's quite normal but it will get easier. What you have read about represents PDPs in a highly developed form, but we all have to start somewhere and in this chapter we discuss how we can avoid drowning by dipping our toe in the water first. Therefore, we will learn how to write an abbreviated PDP and evaluate it. In reality, for all the jargon and concepts that educationists are wont to use, most GPs, having written their first development plan, have little difficulty in coming to terms with the process and they are quickly able to make their PDPs more sophisticated (and useful) in subsequent years. I am sure that this will be your experience too.

The first year

Even though you have this book and could theoretically 'fly solo', it is better to write your first plan as part of a small group. This is because you can share your anxieties with others who are at a similar stage and can help each other by talking about your needs and how they might be addressed. The group may comprise doctors from different practices or from the same practice, and there are pros and cons to both approaches. The former has the benefit of a wider range of experience and possibly of attitudes, and this can encourage GPs to share good practice and become more broad-minded. The latter group benefits from being able to bear the needs of the practice in mind when prioritising the needs of individuals. Doctors in such groups also have a vested interest in making each other's plans successful and this can help the practice to achieve its aims. Some GPs may regard this 'pressure' as being useful whilst others might find it unwelcome – it rather depends on the time management and personalities of those involved. Your GP tutor can facilitate such a group, and in Sheffield groups of up to a dozen GPs are organised to meet three times in the first year. These meetings have the following purposes:

- **First meeting:** to allow each GP to identify at least one educational need and be helped to write it out in the form of a basic PDP. After this meeting, each GP puts together the other learning needs that they have identified at this stage, and writes a plan with the guidance of their GP tutor. Because this plan is the first version for the year, it is called the 'initial personal development plan'.

- **Second meeting:** GPs discuss their progress and in particular the changes (additions and deletions) that they have made to their initial development plan. Again, there is the opportunity to share concerns and ideas

Before the final meeting, the tutor prompts GPs to complete their development plans and to be prepared to discuss the outcome of their learning.

- **Third meeting:** GPs evaluate their final PDP by using a form. In our area the evaluation form is submitted with the development plan, if PGEA is required.

Writing the initial learning plan

In the first meeting, GPs are encouraged to think about their performance. You can do this by giving yourself 10 minutes to answer the following questions. Forms for the exercises discussed are printed at the end of this chapter.

- What three things do I do well?
- What three things do I do badly?

This will help you focus on what you might need to learn.

Next, try filling in the following form as shown below (a blank form is provided on p. 58). Give yourself 10–15 minutes for this task.

What, specifically, do I need to learn?
How to use a personal computer. Specifically, how to use the word processor.

Why do I need to learn this?
Everyone else seems to be more computer literate than me. My partners produce their own practice-related documents but I have to use the secretary, which creates friction within the partnership.

How am I going to learn?
I've heard that there is a book, *Word for Dummies*, which sounds to be at about my level. Also, there is an evening class for beginners at the local college that I could attend.

How will I use this in practice?
I'm due to go on a family planning refresher course soon. I'll use the computer to write up any new developments that I learn about and give each of my partners and the practice nurses a copy – that will surprise them all!

In the time available, you will probably be able to list two or three learning needs and how you would address them.

Now split into groups of two or three and, in turn, each talk through one learning need from your forms. The third question, *How am I going to learn?*, is usually the most important at this stage, as other people can help by suggesting resources that might be available or, better still, ones that are known to be useful. Quite often, GPs offer to help each other by putting colleagues in touch with a resource or even by providing personal support. This is the most valuable part of the meeting and 30–45 minutes should be set aside for it. At the end of this time, you will have had a chance to think through at least one goal and answered all four questions in relation to it, as a result of which, believe it or not, you will have written your first development plan!

Some doctors prefer to continue working through their learning needs in their small groups, as described above. An alternative is to reconvene as a large group and use it to come up with ideas about how to address those learning needs that have proved problematic.

At the close of the meeting, exchange contact details with your colleagues and GP tutor. You are now all set to think about your other learning needs and to write these up in the form of an initial PDP.

What is expected of me?

It is important not to be too ambitious. Each of the learning plans shown in the previous chapter would take many hours to complete. This degree of complexity is certainly not mandatory and particularly in the first year it is more important to get on board with the process of undertaking a simple PDP, than to attempt to make it gold-plated. The object of your plan is to learn something that has the potential to be useful, so it is far better to be realistic about your goals and thereby learn something, than to over stretch yourself and learn nothing. It is particularly pleasing if learning can be applied to practise but we recognise that this cannot always be the case. In years to come, as you become more adept at the process, you will find that you are able to work backwards, selecting some improvements in patient care and determining what skills you will need to obtain in order to bring this about.

When assessing your first attempts at PDPs, most tutors will not be looking for much sophistication, but the following pointers might help you.

- Don't identify too many learning needs in your initial development plan. Two or three are probably enough. This is because working through each goal, even the simplest, always takes longer than anticipated and because so many learning needs that demand urgent attention arise during the course of the year, we need to leave room for some of them in our plans.

- Try to be as specific as possible about what you need to learn, and remember that this should be a *need* and not just a *want*. If you are too general about your needs ('I need to learn more about family planning'), then you are much less likely to succeed than if your aim is more specific ('I need to learn how to fit an IUD').

- Say why the need is worth attending to by stating *how* it became an issue. By doing this you are in effect describing how you assessed your educational needs. If you realise where your need came from, you are also more likely to realise how your new learning will be used. For example, figures might show that you request far more lumbar X-rays than your partners, and you might realise that this is because you feel uncomfortable at managing low back pain. Using this to define your learning need (to learn when X-rays should be requested for low back pain), allows you to manage the condition better and reduce the number of radiology requests.

- When you think about how you intend to learn, try to be a little creative and avoid going to lecture after lecture. This advice is not mandatory as different styles suit different people, but different learning methods also suit different learning needs and you may be restricting your options unnecessarily.

- Even if you are unable to say that you will apply your learning directly to patient care, try to state how your PDP might make you a better practitioner.

Evaluating my first plan

At the end of the year, a simple evaluation will be required which will help to focus your mind on the value of your activities and the implications for your subsequent plan. Here is an example based on the development plan that you saw earlier. A blank form is included at the end of this chapter.

Which were the most valuable learning activities and why?
Attending the evening class. I felt relieved that there were others in the same boat, some even less confident than I was. The teaching was not too technical and we all had computer terminals to work on, so the sessions were very practical.

Which were the least valuable learning activities and why?
I found that reading about Word 97 was rather dull. The book I chose was written for an American audience, and I found it irritating. In my view, nothing beats hands-on experience with the computer.

In what ways have you been able to apply your learning in practice?
I did what I set out to do and presented my first word-processed document to my partners after the family planning update, and received a gratifying response. This has spurred me on to use the computer more, producing updates of our menopause clinic and travel clinic protocols.

What learning needs might you wish to carry forward to your next portfolio?
Now that I have a basic understanding, I should like to use the Internet, particularly for e-mail.

Summary

I hope you now feel that your first PDP is within your grasp. Your GP tutor will advise as to the standards that are expected in your region, and you will not be unsupported in your attempts to get started. You will find as time goes on that you will use more of the ideas and techniques you have read about in the preceding chapters, as a result of which your learning will become more focused and more effective. However, first things first. Why not have a go at writing your PDP and discover for yourself why those who use them would not go back to old-fashioned CME.

What three things do I do well?

1

2

3

What three things do I do badly?

1

2

3

Initial PDP

What, specifically, do I need to learn?

Why do I need to learn this?

How am I going to learn?

How will I use this in practice?

Evaluation form

Which were the most valuable learning activities and why?

Which were the least valuable learning activities and why?

In what ways have you been able to apply your learning in practice?

What learning needs might you wish to carry forward to your next portfolio?

5 Assessing PDPs

Key points

- PDPs are not plans in isolation, but are part of a continuing learning spiral.
- Evaluating the PDP helps to make future learning more effective and this evaluation can be based on the assessment of certain criteria.
- The purpose of assessment is *not* to make pass/fail decisions.
- Assessment of the criteria provides observations that can be used to further the professional development of the GP.
- These criteria can be used by GPs for self-evaluation, or by others such as GP tutors who have responsibility for assisting their colleagues with their PDPs.
- A template can be used to help GPs make progress with the sophistication of their learning.
- Assessment of the PDP process by the GP provides useful feedback and helps to keep the focus of education where it belongs – on the learner.

Introduction

In the previous two chapters we looked at the principles underlying the PDP, saw examples of sophisticated development plans and learned how to make a sound start. GP tutors provide support for the PDP process and offer constructive criticism with the aim of helping us to make our learning more effective. To do this, they have to make judgements or 'assessments' on our approach to learning and in this chapter we will look at the basis on which such assessments can be made. No one likes the word assessment but it is the purpose that is important and I should emphasise that we are not talking about making pass/fail decisions. Rather, the aim is to make observations designed to encourage reflection and change, and in this chapter there will be the opportunity to make such observations on examples derived from real-life PDPs. In doing so, readers can learn to evaluate their own plans or to comment on their colleagues' plans if they have the responsibility for doing so. An interactive approach is used and I would suggest that this chapter is best read when some personal experience of writing and implementing a PDP has been gained. Let us begin by looking at the background to the assessment process.

PDPs have been widely adopted by GPs across the UK and, although not compulsory, they have become the favoured route for gaining PGEA in a number of regions. The experience of both learners and GP tutors is that this new approach to postgraduate education is successful because it is learner-centred, flexible and feasible. PDPs are being developed in an age of increasing accountability where the mechanism and content of a doctor's learning are matters of public interest, and this is bringing several influences to bear on the PDP process.

First, Revalidation is likely to require that doctors:

- Have an awareness of their learning needs.
- Use educational activities appropriate to meet those needs.
- Produce changes in clinical practice as a result of their learning.

PDPs will probably be a compulsory requirement for Revalidation, and it therefore seems sensible to ensure that those doctors who use them, construct them in a way that meets these requirements.

Second, external agents such as revalidators and appraisers may wish to see proof of a GP's commitment to lifelong learning. Because of this, doctors will want to use their PDP to demonstrate such commitment and the paperwork supporting the PDP process should be capable of providing this proof. The bureaucracy associated with the PDP will necessarily be greater than was required for PGEA alone, but it will now serve four purposes.

1 Help to navigate the learner through the four stages of the PDP cycle, namely planning, implementation, amendment and evaluation.
2 Provide proof of activity for PGEA purposes.
3 Provide evidence of learning when required for purposes such as Revalidation or appraisal.
4 Provide information by which the GP tutor can assist the learner to develop professionally.

Third, and leading on from the last point, GP tutors will have to consider how the information contained in the PDP can and should be used. Chief amongst tutors' considerations is the fact that the contents of the doctor's PDP have been entrusted to them to be discussed jointly with the GP, and to be used with benign intent. With the exception of very rare situations where matters of serious under performance or professional misconduct become evident, tutors have a duty to use this information confidentially unless wider discussion has been agreed by the learner.

Bearing these points in mind, how then can the PDP and its attendant paperwork be assessed in a way that meets these expectations? In this chapter, we will first describe the PDP spiral and the elements within it and then work through examples, presented as *Checkpoints*. Each example provides a focus for constructive criticism but is presented in isolation of any other knowledge of the learner, their previous learning, working practices, etc., all of which would have a bearing on the advice that might be given. To derive the maximum benefit, I suggest that you make no assumptions about the learner and offer your own observations before comparing these with the comments at the end of the chapter. Because these are not pass/fail judgements, the comments provided should not be regarded as 'answers', although they do represent a consensus view of GP tutors in North Trent.

The PDP spiral

PDPs should not be thought of as a written plan in isolation, but as part of a process. Let us imagine that we are starting from scratch, in which case the process is as follows:

- Construction of the initial development plan for Year 1.
- Implementation of the plan, including the collection of evidence for the portfolio.
- Amendment of the learning needs in the light of changing priorities.
- Evaluation of the completed plan.
- Construction of the initial development plan for Year 2, etc.

I use the word 'spiral' rather than 'cycle' to emphasise that with every completed turn of the PDP wheel, we are further on in our educational development than we were at the same point in the preceding year. This is a crucial point because, as we will see later, our completed development plan should be able to demonstrate educational *progress*, particularly with regard to improvements in patient care.

To get a feel for the PDP spiral, let us look at each of the elements in more detail.

Construction of the initial development plan for Year 1

This involves sitting down and writing a plan that comprises a short list of usually two or three educational needs. Each of these needs is then sketched out in terms of how they might be met and what evidence might be kept for the portfolio to prove that we have undertaken the planned learning.

Implementation of the plan, including the collection of evidence for the portfolio

Work can begin straight away on attending to our stated priorities. By implementation, we mean undertaking the learning activities that we have decided to use, be they reading, being taught a new skill, etc. This doesn't mean that we have to stick to the methods stated in our initial plan as we may find that other activities become available that prove to be more appropriate. These activities will give rise to some documentary proof of learning such as our written evaluation of them, and this may be used as evidence to be kept in our portfolio.

Amendment of the learning needs in the light of changing priorities

During the year priorities will change. For instance, a learning need may prove difficult to meet because of lack of resources, or a new practice priority may result in our educational needs being directed elsewhere. Amendments are therefore not only 'allowed' but they are inevitable and necessary.

Evaluation of the completed plan

GP tutors consider evaluation to be an essential part of the process as through it doctors can learn valuable lessons from the success or otherwise of their development plan. This allows future learning to be better targeted and pitfalls that have led to failure in meeting our objectives to be avoided.

Construction of the initial development plan for Year 2

Leading on from the evaluation and possibly as part of the same meeting, we can begin to plan the following year's plan whilst learning the lessons from the previous one.

Support can be provided throughout the educational year, but assessment can occur at different points within it. For example, in North Trent assessment occurs when the initial development plan is written and again at the end of the year when the completed plan is submitted for assessment. We will now consider the principles by which we could assess initial plans, any amendments made and the completed plan.

The initial development plan

The initial plan comprises a few educational needs, each of which can be written out as shown in the following example (Table 5.1). This illustration is an exemplar rather than being indicative of the first attempts of most GPs.

Table 5.1: Initial development plan

No.	Educational need	Reason for inclusion in development plan	Learning objectives	Activities to be used	What evidence will you keep?
1	Learn how to manage osteoporosis in patients on long-term steroids.	Significant event: I had a patient on long-term steroids who suffered a vertebral fracture.	1 Know how to identify the at-risk group. 2 Know how to prevent osteoporosis in this group. 3 Know how to treat existing patients with osteoporosis in line with best practice.	Read recent literature: journal articles and existing guidelines. Speak to colleagues in the metabolic bone unit.	1 Summarise key points from my reading. 2 Produce practice guidelines. 3 Produce an audit of osteoporosis management.

The layout of the plan may not match the paperwork in your area, but all such plans should include the three mandatory elements from Revalidation, namely the educational need, how it might be met and what evidence will be kept to show that learning has taken place.

To see how each of these elements can be assessed, let us look in detail at the headings from the example shown.

Number

In some regions such as North Trent the PDP is linked to PGEA, with up to 30 hours' accreditation being available for the completed plan, and it comes as a surprise to many GPs to see how quickly the hours can accumulate. Generally, meeting about five learning needs is sufficient to produce 30 hours' activity for the year. At the time that the initial development plan is written, we need only plan two or three needs in the manner prescribed. This is because some learning needs fall by the wayside, perhaps because they are not feasible, and other needs will surface in response to clinical practice and the demands of practice life. Knowing this, it is helpful to build in sufficient flexibility for these amendments to occur.

Educational need/reason for inclusion in the development plan

- **The educational need is of relevance to primary care**

The PDP is first and foremost a *personal* development plan and although it may be influenced by external factors it should be owned and controlled by the learner. The PDP must reflect learning in the context of primary care and, broadly speaking, this means that whatever the GP is proposing to learn about should have the potential of improving the care that the doctor provides and/or of helping them to develop professionally.

Needs do not have to be *directly* applicable to patient care and this is important because much learning results in a change of knowledge or attitude that may only later lead to a change in behaviour that can be demonstrated.

Learning within primary care can and should be broad-based. Hence, it is just as appropriate for GPs to learn about the use of homeopathy or medical ethics as it is to update themselves on diabetic management. Likewise, learning needs are not always clinical, as patient care may be improved as much by better service delivery as by the use of biomedical knowledge.

- **There is a balance between the learning needs**

Meaning that there is a balance between:

- The learner's agenda derived from their role as a GP and other posts that they might hold, as well as the wider needs of the practice and of the locality.
- Learning that might merely inform and learning that has an immediate practical application to patient care.
- Learning needs that fulfil the Red Book requirements (health promotion, disease management and service management) if PGEA is being claimed.

Checkpoint 1

Based on this, what thoughts do you have about the plan shown in Table 5.2? For this exercise, assume that this is the totality of the learner's PDP.

Table 5.2: Initial development plan

No.	Educational need	Reason for inclusion in development plan	Learning objectives	Activities to be used	What evidence will you keep?
1	Learn about sports medicine.	I wish to undertake a MSc.			
2	Develop leadership skills.	I have a role on the PCT board that involves leading my colleagues.			
3	Learn about modern partnership agreements.	We are due to appoint a new partner this year and our current agreement is 10 years old.			
4	Keep up to date by reading the journals.	There is a need to practise evidence-based medicine.			

Table 5.3: Initial development plan

No.	Educational need	Reason for inclusion in development plan	Learning objectives	Activities to be used	What evidence will you keep?
1	Become a trainer.	The existing trainer in the practice is retiring.			
2	Learn the new guidelines for cervical cytology call/recall.	The clinic is run by the practice nurse, and my knowledge of the guidelines is rusty.			
3	HRT update.	As the female partner, patients who require HRT come to me for advice.			

- The 'need' represents a deficiency

Is the learner addressing a need or a want, i.e. are they attending to a deficiency or purely satisfying an interest? The two are not incompatible and, indeed, even if GPs have identified something that they need to learn about, they have to want to address this need if they are to successfully complete their plan.

Checkpoint 2

The very act of undertaking a PDP encourages doctors to look more closely at their needs. Looking at the reasons for inclusion in the development plan helps to gauge both the degree of need and the motivation for learning. With this in mind, what comments do you have about the examples shown in Table 5.3?

Looking back at Table 5.1 we can see that the doctor identified a need through a significant event, and these events are influential (because they are often emotive) in producing change. The use of significant events to drive the PDP, particularly when they are derived from adverse patient consequences, is important as they often indicate genuine educational need.

- There is evidence of need

By evidence, we mean both subjective measures derived from reflection, questionnaires and feedback, and objective measures such as audit, surveys and significant event analyses. Evidence of this sort is not compulsory but as GPs become more advanced with planning their learning, it is likely that a short description of how educational needs have been derived will become more commonplace.

- If the GP has a specialised role, this is being considered

Some GPs have particular responsibilities by virtue of their role as teachers, researchers or GPs with a special interest, undertaking such posts as clinical assistantships. For these doctors, there may be a need (e.g. because of appraisal and Revalidation) to demonstrate that part of their continuing education is devoted to maintaining skills in these non-generalist areas. The GP tutor might discuss whether the learner wishes to demonstrate such training and education through their PDP.

- Addressing the need appears feasible

For the learning plan to be successful it is important that it is not over-ambitious, as the plan is not a record of *all* the learning in which the GP is engaged, but only that part of it that they wish to have accredited. An assessment of the feasibility of the plan can be made by looking at the workload represented by the plan and the resources required by it. The workload can be gauged by looking at how ambitious the objectives seem to be and the resources can be inferred by examining the proposed activities. For example, some activities such as courses may seem like a good idea but may not be available, accessible or affordable.

Meeting the educational need: learning objectives and activities to be used

- The learning objectives are SMART

Having appropriate learning objectives is not a sterile academic exercise designed to frustrate the learner, but is fundamental to success in the PDP spiral. Objectives define the desired outcomes of the learning process; there may be only one if the educational need is small or there may be several if the need is larger and has to be broken down into a number of manageable steps.

In practice, objectives often state the new ability that the learner is seeking to acquire. Table 5.1 gives examples of objectives that define smaller areas of new *knowledge* that the learner needs in order to meet his overall educational need. Sometimes, the objective may refer to a practical *skill*, e.g. 'to be able to fit GyneFix IUCD', or an *attitude* such as 'to understand what teenagers want from our family planning services'. Whatever the objective, being specific about it is the most important feature.

Checkpoint 3

What comments would you make about the objectives in Table 5.4?

- Appropriate activities are used

At the time that the initial learning plan is written, the exact activities to be used may not be clear and will almost certainly change as learning proceeds. It is

Table 5.4: Initial development plan

No.	Educational need	Reason for inclusion in development plan	Learning objectives	Activities to be used	What evidence will you keep?
1	Learn the UKPDS guidelines.	I'm concerned that my diabetic patients may not be adequately managed.	Feel more confident about how to manage Type 2 diabetes.		
2	Investigate how feasible it is to become a paperless practice.	Many practices are doing this, and our paper records are becoming unwieldy.	Talk with a colleague who has made the change.		
3	To improve my management of patients with terminal illness.	As a new GP, I feel that I lack experience in this area.	Undertake a case review of the next such patient that I treat.		

important that the initial learning plan shows that the learner has some idea about how they would start to learn, the priority being that their chosen activities seem appropriate to the stated objectives.

Activities are otherwise known as 'learning methods', and as a secondary issue we might look at the range of methods being used. Some learners prefer to work in isolation or learn passively by reading or going to lectures. However, as postgraduate education becomes increasingly multidisciplinary we might wish to think about using interactive activities such as talking to colleagues, working in groups or using team-based approaches.

Checkpoint 4

Look at the activities in the learning plan shown in Table 5.5. To what degree do they reflect these principles?

Collecting the evidence

The principles of adult learning are not new to GPs, but the collection of evidence to serve the purpose of accountability is a recent requirement. Here is a summary of the points made about the proof of learning in Chapter 3.

- **There is evidence of learning and sometimes evidence of application**

In its most basic form, evidence may be proof that the learner has engaged in educational activity. Beyond this, there may be evidence of reflective learning perhaps through a learning log or evaluation form. Finally, there may be evidence of learning that has been applied to practice.

- **Evidence arises from mainstream activity**

The most useful evidence is that which helps the learner to get the most from their educational activity as well as serving the needs of accountability, and this may include guidelines, protocols and audits.

- **Quality, not quantity**

Lengthy summaries of the content of articles are not required, as what is useful to the learner is not the whole content but the parts of it that are new to him. Hence,

Table 5.5: Initial development plan

No.	Educational need	Reason for inclusion in development plan	Learning objectives	Activities to be used	What evidence will you keep?
1	Improve my management of mild asthma.	British Thoracic Society guidelines have been revised. My management may not be in line with them.	Know when to introduce asthma prophylaxis.	Go to a lecture given by the chest physician.	
2	Improve my treatment of the painful shoulder.	My management options are limited, as I am not confident about injecting the joint.	Know how to inject the shoulder joint.	Look at some photographs on injection technique.	
3	Learn how to use the practice computer.	The computer in my consulting room has been updated. My partners seem to be experts, but I feel ignorant about using a PC.	To be able to use the Internet, particularly for email.

To be able to use the word processor. | Enrol in a distance-learning course that teaches computer skills. | |

considerable time spent reading may be summarised in only a few sentences and this may surprise or even disappoint the learner, who might be expecting to keep reams of material. The resulting portfolio may not look so impressive in terms of sheer bulk, but GPs should be reassured that quality not quantity is the key.

- **Certificates of learning**

Occasionally, certificates are issued that do in themselves confirm that learning has taken place. Examples include certification that a doctor has been trained in a particular skill (e.g. fitting an IUCD), certificates of satisfactory completion of distance-learning courses and diplomas and degrees awarded by educational bodies. All of these are valid forms of evidence, but if doctors are engaged in certified forms of learning, they should not feel that they have to obtain the relevant end-point certificate in order to demonstrate learning, as learning occurs throughout.

Intermediate goals can be set and appropriate evidence collected. For example, a doctor studying for a homeopathy diploma could set a lower challenge and therefore more achievable goal related to the use of homeopathic remedies in treating musculo-ligamentous disorders. Hence, instead of waiting for the diploma, he could, for example, use his anonymised case notes as evidence.

Checkpoint 5

Consider the evidence in Table 5.6. How appropriate do you feel it is and what suggestions would you make to the learner?

Amending the learning plan

We have previously seen how the PDP provides an opportunity to be proactive with our learning. However, because the plan is written at the start of the year we will not know if the priorities defined in the initial development plan will maintain their importance throughout the year. Our priorities may change, perhaps prompted by practice or locality demands or by significant events relating to clinical care. In addition, our original learning needs may have to be deferred because the resources required to meet them (lectures, courses, etc.) are not available. Therefore, we may wish to change our plan, and such amendments

Table 5.6: Initial development plan

No.	Educational need	Reason for inclusion in development plan	Learning objectives	Activities to be used	What evidence will you keep?
1	Learn about 'bleed-free' HRT.	My menopausal patients have been asking about it.	Know the preparations that I could prescribe.	Sit in at the menopause clinic.	A log of the dates of attendance, signed by the clinic doctor.
			Know the indications for their use.		
2	Update myself on the treatment of heart failure in primary care.	Old drugs are finding a new lease of life. How should I use them?	Know which drugs I can initiate and how to do so.	Read a recent series of articles on heart failure from the *BMJ*.	Photocopies of the articles that I have read.
3	To pass the MRCGP.	I need the qualification in order to become a trainer.	Know the factual material required.	Read the medical journals.	MRCGP diploma.
			Be able to demonstrate consulting skills.	Revise from the textbooks.	
				Attend a course.	
				Practice video consultations.	

(additions and deletions) are not only 'allowed' but are inevitable and demonstrate the responsiveness of our learning to the context of our working lives.

Being aware of the need to allow for flexibility in the plan means that we do not commit ourselves to a large number of learning needs at the start of the year. For example, some GPs like to learn from needs that are identified in the consultation and therefore allow time in their annual plan, e.g. a quarter of their accredited hours, to make use of these opportunities.

We will have put a lot of thought into writing our initial plan, and if we are to make wholesale changes it will be important to make sure that the integrity of the plan is not compromised. We could do this by asking the following questions about the amendments.

1 Are educational needs that we considered important (e.g. on the basis of objective assessment such as audit) being abandoned?

2 Is there an obstacle to learning, such as a resource or training issue, that could be addressed?

3 Is the balance of the plan, as discussed earlier, being compromised? If so, does this matter?

4 Is the amended plan feasible in the given timescale?

5 Will the plan still meet the needs of Revalidation/PGEA?

Therefore, although amendments can be freely made, we should be prepared to justify them if required. To make this easier, the PDP paperwork could include a page for amendments such as that shown in Table 5.7.

Checkpoint 6

We have previously looked at how to comment on additions to the learning plan and therefore we will now take the opportunity to look at examples of deletions from the plan. Examining these, what thoughts do you have about them and what might you suggest to the learner?

Table 5.7: Personal development plan: amendments

Educational need	Reason for including/ removing from development plan	Learning objectives for additions	Activities to be used for additions	What evidence will you keep?
To understand why some of my patients are being over-treated with thyroxine.	I removed this need in order to look at our chiropody services.			
To be able to use the word processor.	This was removed because the book that came with the PC was not very helpful.			

Evaluating the learning process

In many regions, the PDP is a route by which GPs achieve their PGEA. If this is the case for the learner, one aim of assessment at the end of the educational year is to confirm that the work submitted meets the PGEA requirements. This is achieved by looking at the doctor's log of activity for each learning need and checking that the hours seem plausible and are appropriate for the category claimed.

From an educational perspective, the more important evaluation is that of the learning process, which consists of determining whether:

- The methods of identifying learning needs were discussed.
- The learning objectives were evaluated.
- The usefulness of learning methods was evaluated.
- The learning outcomes were evaluated.
- Learning needs arising from the reflective process were discussed.
- The learner provided feedback on the PDP process.

As we can see, the emphasis is on encouraging reflection with the aim of making future learning more effective. Each of the principles in the list above has been elaborated upon in Chapter 3 (pp 39–41). Look at this section again and then comment on the self-completed evaluation shown in Checkpoint 7. What might you wish to discuss with the learner?

Making progress

We have seen that the PDP comprises several elements, each of which can be addressed at differing degrees of complexity. To look at how we can progress from basic to sophisticated levels with our PDPs over the years, it is useful to have a guide and the Appendix on p. 89 shows one approach that could be used. In practice, no one performs at the same level for each of these elements and it can be encouraging to newcomers to see that even though they may seem to be basic in some areas, they may be more advanced in others.

Checkpoint 7

Personal development plan: evaluation

- **How did you identify your learning needs for this PDP, and what other methods might you include in your next PDP?**

Mostly by making a note of situations that make me uneasy. This works well for me, but I could look at my referral rates next time.

- **Which objectives were easiest to achieve and why?**

Learning how to fit the Mirena coil, because I had good tuition and practical experience at the local FPA clinic.

- **Which objectives were most difficult to achieve and why?**

Mental health, because the subject is so large and the methods (*see* below) didn't help.

- **Which were the most valuable learning activities and why?**

The distance-learning package on ophthalmology, because I could do it in my own time.

- **Which were the least valuable learning activities and why?**

Attending a team meeting on mental health. It was not constructive, and we spent most of the time bickering about who saw the most number of depressed patients!

- **In what ways have you been able to apply your learning in practice?**

I feel more confident at treating the red eye correctly.

- **What benefits to your patients do you feel have occurred as a result of your learning?**

My patients have probably benefited from better management of the red eye, but I could not prove it.

- **Are there any learning needs that you wish to carry forward to your next PDP?**

I'm still not sure what exactly we are supposed to do as GPs regarding the NSF in mental health.

- **Do you have any suggestions or comments about the administration of your PDP or the support that you have received?**

The support was great. The paperwork was a chore and I would have preferred to submit my forms by computer.

Summary

The following represents a short summary of the assessment principles discussed in this chapter and could be used as a checklist when evaluating the PDP.

Initial learning plan

Educational need/reason for inclusion

1   The educational need is of relevance to primary care.

2   There is a balance between the learning needs.

As guided by:

- personal agenda
- personal contribution to practice development, e.g. as guided by clinical governance
- the potential to directly improve patient care
- the requirements of PGEA.

3   **The need represents a deficiency.**

Guided by the reasons for inclusion in the development plan and whether this is a need or purely a want.

4   **There is evidence of need.**

Thereby encouraging learners to use the subjective and objective techniques of self-assessment, such as reflection, feedback, audit, data analysis, etc.

5   **If the GP has a specialised role, this is being considered.**

Although not a requirement for the PDP, if the GP is a teacher/researcher/clinical assistant, etc. they may wish to incorporate learning related to this in their plan.

6   **Addressing the need appears feasible.**

Some needs are very large and may need to be refined. Looking at the needs overall, the workload involved in meeting the objectives should not be prohibitive and the resources should be available.

Learning objectives

The learning objectives are SMART.

The objectives are derived from the stated learning needs, thereby helping the learner to know when the end-point has been reached.

Activities to be used

Appropriate activities are used.

The activities are appropriate to the objectives. Where appropriate, issues concerning the range of activities and the use of interactive or group methods can be discussed.

Collecting the evidence

'Good' evidence might be illustrated by the following:

1   There is evidence of learning and sometimes evidence of application.

Where possible, learners should be encouraged to collect evidence that indicates that learning has taken place. To meet the needs of Revalidation there should be periodic evidence of the application of learning to practice in a way that benefits patients.

2   Evidence arises from mainstream activity.

Wherever possible, evidence should derive from documentation that GPs would be planning to produce for their own use, e.g. aide-mémoire to use in surgery, new or revised practice protocols, etc. In this way, duplication of effort can be avoided.

3   There is evidence of reflective learning.

Meaning that rather than collect primary material such as journal articles, learners could highlight the relevant points, produce bullet points or brief evaluations of what they have learned from reading, attending meetings or courses, etc. The key point is that keeping medical literature or certificates of attendance is not in itself proof of learning.

4   Certificates of learning.

Some forms of certification (diplomas, successful completion of distance learning, etc.) *are* proof of learning and are therefore appropriate.

Amendments to the learning plan

Learners could consider whether changes to the plan are appropriate along the following lines.

1 Are educational needs that are considered important being abandoned?
2 Is there an obstacle to learning, such as a resource or training issue that could be addressed?
3 Is the balance of the plan, as discussed earlier, being compromised? If so, does this matter?
4 Is the amended plan feasible in the given timescale?
5 Will the plan still meet the needs of Revalidation/PGEA?

Evaluation of the learning process

From the completed evaluation form, the following criteria could be assessed.

1 The learning objectives were evaluated.
2 The usefulness of learning methods was evaluated.
3 The learning outcomes were evaluated.
4 Learning needs arising from the reflective process were discussed.
5 The learner provided feedback on the PDP process.

Checkpoint comments

Checkpoint 1

- The plan seems almost entirely doctor-centred in that there are no activities that relate directly to practice-based goals such as clinical governance activities.

- With regard to improved patient care, the link with learning is present but is not strong. In encouraging the learner to expand on his reasons for choosing these educational needs, a connection between learning and patient care might be found. If this were the case, the learner could be encouraged to consider objectives that focused on clinical management, e.g. 'Improving the treatment for patients presenting with sports injuries'. Alternatively, the learner might add another need that specifically targeted clinical care.

- Undertaking a degree or diploma is not an uncommon activity, and is appropriate for inclusion in the PDP. However, to achieve balance we need to be careful about activities that might dominate the plan, and higher learning of this sort can threaten to do so because of its very large content. A reasonable compromise, because such learning can take several years, would be to include elements from it in successive PDPs. Alternatively, it could be agreed that one educational need will consume most of the current plan with the proviso that the following year's PDP will be more balanced.

- The need to keep up to date is not in question – all doctors are required to do this. However, the purpose of the initial plan is to show how we will meet our disclosed deficiencies. Stating that we will read the journals does not show that we have recognised a particular need, nor does it guarantee that we will learn anything! It is better to wait until we become aware through our reading that there is a deficiency to be addressed, and then incorporate this need as a later addition to our plan.

- If this was the *entire* PDP and we were claiming PGEA we might run into accreditation problems, as it seems that health promotion and disease management may be poorly represented.

Checkpoint 2

- In the first example, the GP needs to become a trainer, but who is this driven by? It could be that the practice requires someone to replace the outgoing trainer and the GP has been persuaded to take on this role. Even though becoming a trainer would greatly help the GP to develop, for such a large undertaking it would be important to verify the learner's commitment.

- In the second example, the learner states that the cervical cytology service has been devolved to the practice nurse. Why then does he feel that *he* also needs to learn the new guidelines? The use of the word 'rusty' implies that he has recognised a deficiency, but perhaps in a multidisciplinary team it might be more appropriate for the nurse rather than the doctor to keep up to date with the guidelines, and for the doctor to know whom to turn to for help in this area when required.

- In the final example, several factors emerge. The learner may be an inexperienced GP, be responding to a significant event or have accepted responsibility for providing this service, in which case the need is appropriate. We may consider whether, if she is already expert on the use of HRT, obtaining an HRT update is attending to the most pressing of her learning needs. Also, the fact that female patients are coming to this doctor *might* mean that other members of the team are not providing an adequate service. This topic would need sensitive discussion!

Checkpoint 3

- The first learning objective seems rather vague. Feeling more confident is an outcome that would apply to most learning needs, but it is not a specific objective. It does not indicate what *ability*, rather than feeling, the learner is seeking to achieve and gives no indication of how he would know when he had achieved his objective. In practice, how would the doctor know when he was 'confident enough' and how valid is this as an end-point of learning? Unfortunately, competence decays far more quickly than confidence!

  If SMART objectives are not set, there is the risk that the learner would take far longer to reach their destination, or worse still go off track and miss it entirely, leaving them with feelings of disappointment and frustration.

  It is important to be honest, and admitting to large areas of 'weakness' is a valuable first step that should be encouraged. This could serve as a foundation and the process of setting specific objectives could then be used to help refine the area of diabetic management that needs prioritising. In the first example, it might transpire that learning about optimising the control of blood sugar, blood pressure or attendance for routine retinoscopy might be the main areas of anxiety, and each of these could then be written as appropriate objectives.

- In the second example, the objective 'talk with a colleague' is not SMART and is really an activity or learning method rather than an objective. The idea of talking to someone who has had experience of the proposed change is perfectly sensible, but it would help learning to be more effective and time-efficient if the learner could decide in advance what their main concerns were in relation to becoming paperless. On the basis of this, the doctor could then decide what issues he wished to raise with his colleague. For example, he might want to talk about the resources required to become paperless, the logistics of change, medico-legal aspects, confidentiality, how records are made available for visits, and so on. Each of these would make a suitable objective and the discussion, when it occurred, would have more chance of being productive.

- In the last example, 'undertake a case review' is again an activity rather than a learning objective. If this was our development plan, we might think about what we were hoping to gain from this activity and this could suggest certain standards in palliative care that we might wish to measure ourselves against. Conversely, the process of reflection might indicate that we were not sure what those standards should be. In either event, we would have the basis for establishing some clearer objectives by which we could meet our overall aim of improving our management of patients with terminal illness.

Checkpoint 4

- The first two activities lack a clear potential for interactive learning and this is an issue that could be raised. It might be that the learner prefers to work alone, but it may be that he feels insecure or isolated.

  The first activity is the traditional lecture given by a secondary care specialist. These are often popular as the lecture format is familiar and feels safe. The learner may also feel that what he needs to learn can be told to him by an expert. This may be true but looking at the learner's need, which is to improve the management of *mild* asthma, we might question how appropriate it was to be seeking the views of specialists who probably never see the condition described.

  The lecture could be made more relevant to a GP audience by including a primary care resource such as a GP or nurse with expertise in asthma, or by providing some focus on asthma presentations in primary care.

- The second activity seems rather passive for the acquisition of such a practical skill. If the learner is already expert in injecting other joints, then reading about a new technique may be appropriate. However, for the novice using a book is unlikely to be as effective as being shown how to give the injection. It would help to explore why the learner had chosen this activity rather than other methods, such as learning from a colleague or attending a clinical skills course. It might be that they feel inadequate or fear being embarrassed, both of which are important issues to explore sensitively before commenting on the choice of activity or suggesting alternatives such as those described.

- Some of the same comments apply to the third activity. The learner has expressed his feelings of inadequacy compared to his partners, and may feel that they would not be suitable teachers. This could be discussed and hopefully overcome, as GPs are often happy to help their colleagues in this way. In general, many distance-learning courses are of high-quality, especially in this computer age, and such a course might be appropriate for this learner. The learner stated that his need was in relation to the use of the practice computer, and we might check with them that the content of the course was addressing this need, rather than being a general course on the use of computers. Many practices have a nominated Information Technology Lead, and this could be an opportunity to learn from a team member. Alternatively, the supplier of the practice computers might be prepared to offer tuition. In sharing ideas in this way we might find that a particular learning need is common to several people, in which case organising tuition for a group may be a useful next step, and one with which the GP tutor could help.

Checkpoint 5

- For the first need, a log of dates is merely proof of attendance. Better evidence could relate back to the learning objectives and might include an aide-mémoire, such as short notes or a flow chart showing HRT preparations and their indications that could be used in future consultations, or an evaluation of the clinic attendances themselves.

- In the second need, photocopies are not as useful as highlighted text or bullet points. One method is to cite the reference and then make a note of the key points.

- The third need, however laudable, is very ambitious and rather than set such a high target, the learner could think of another that lies en route to the ultimate goal. For example, the learner could decide to improve consulting skills, in which case the evidence might be an assessment of a videotaped consultation carried out by the doctor on his own or in conjunction with a peer who is familiar with this technique, such as a GP trainer.

Checkpoint 6

- For the first deletion, the concern is that the original educational need seemed significant in terms of patient care, or in this case, patient harm. The GP indicates that the need arises from a continuing problem. Each patient found to be over-treated should be regarded as a significant event and if nothing were done, there might be the risk of actual harm. Therefore, although chiropody services might well be important, we might wish to check that this concern was not being overlooked.

- With the second deletion, it is clear that the GP found that his learning method was inadequate for the task. Perhaps another approach such as learning from a colleague or attending a workshop might be better. Alternatively, the learner may feel insecure about using the computer and would prefer to back-pedal on his commitment. Improving IT skills is a very common learning need and being taught by someone who is not an expert but a recent novice can help to build confidence.

- Sometimes, as possibly in the second example, the learner may decide that the learning need still requires attention but needs to be approached in a different way. In that case, tackling the subject could be deferred perhaps to the next PDP.

Checkpoint 7

- The learner shows insight by recognising a form of needs assessment (a log of uneasy situations) that works well for him and by thinking of broadening his repertoire by using objective tools such as the analysis of referrals.

- SMART objectives are the cornerstone of achieving success in the PDP. Perhaps the reason that the family planning objective was successful was because it was clearly focused and directed the GP to a learning method that was appropriate.

- Learners are also encouraged to reflect on whether *lack* of success was related to poor objectives. In this case, the doctor recognises that his objective regarding mental health may have been too large and non-specific to focus his learning.

- The distance-learning package was valued because of its flexibility, but what about its content? Increased confidence was reported, but was this due to the use of this package or to some other factor? Given that the main improvement in skill was related to a limited area of care (managing the red eye), it could be that the ophthalmology package was more comprehensive than was needed. If so, the importance of defining appropriate objectives at the outset of learning is highlighted.

- The least valuable activity was the team meeting, which is a concern because the GP may feel less inclined to use this important activity in the future. Meetings of this sort can be kept on-track through the use of clear objectives, good organisation and chairmanship, etc. There may be other reasons why the meeting was poor, for example the team itself might be dysfunctional or mental health may be an area that is poorly managed by the whole practice, and these issues might need to be explored.

- A heartening feature is that learning has not only been applied to practice, but has probably produced an improvement in patient care. It might be possible to translate a feeling of increased confidence into *evidence* of benefit by analysing referrals, possibly showing a reduction in number or an improvement in the preliminary GP assessment.

- It appears that the learning need in mental health has yet to be addressed, and if this need were carried forward, it would be important to make sure that the learning methods (particularly teamwork) were more likely to be successful next time around.

- The feedback on the PDP process is useful and helps to modify the approach and keep it user-friendly. In response to comments such as this one, paperwork could be made available in electronic form and tutors could communicate with learners by email.

Appendix
PDPs: Making progress

PDP element	Level of sophistication		
	Basic	Intermediate (Additional to basic criteria)	Advanced (Additional to intermediate criteria)
Learning needs	1 Needs are relevant to primary care. 2 Learning needs are expressed as specific learning objectives.	3 Some learning needs are practice-related. 4 Some learning needs are drawn from subjective assessments (e.g. significant events or feedback).	5 Some learning needs are derived from objective assessments (e.g. audit or data analysis).
Method of learning	1 Methods chosen are appropriate to the learning objectives.	2 Some methods chosen are practice-based.	3 Some methods chosen are interactive.
Evidence	1 There is documentary proof of reflective[a] learning. [a] evaluation following attending a lecture, reading an article, etc.	2 There is documentary proof of task-orientated[b] learning. [b] writing a protocol, acquiring a skill, etc.	3 The evidence indicates the influence of new learning on thought or behaviour, e.g. through a commentary or through audit.
Application	1 There is evidence of learning, even if it has not been applied.	2 A change in practice has been reported but not demonstrated.	3 There is evidence of a change in practice.
Self-evaluation	1 The success of the objectives and learning activities is commented upon.	2 Reasons for lack of application of learning/lack of patient benefit are discussed.	3 There is evidence of having learned from the evaluation process.

6 PUNs & DENs©

What are PUNs & DENs?

How can individuals use them?

How do we use PUNs & DENs in our consultations?

How could the practice team use PUNs & DENs?

Summary

Obtaining logbooks

Key points

- The PUNs & DENs approach is self-directed, and is usually based on the consultation.
- It is derived directly from what we do.
- Although it quickly highlights deficiencies, we should also remember our strengths.
- Not all PUNs lead to DENs.
- PUNs can be established more widely, for example through audit.
- Involving others makes the process less subjective, increases its value and makes it more fun!
- Collating the PUNs of individuals allows the Team Educational Needs to be established.

What are PUNs & DENs?

Dr Richard Eve first described PUNs & DENs as a mechanism by which doctors can identify their educational needs by analysing their activity in consultation. His idea was that many of our clinical encounters result in a patient's needs not being met. Some of these *Patient Unmet Needs* (PUNs) may be due to the doctor's lack of knowledge or skill, and identifying them allows us to define the *Doctors Educational Needs* (DENs). What appears below is a variation of the approach described by Dr Eve and appears with his permission.

We've all had the experience in surgery – sometimes several times a day – of thinking 'I must go and look that up'. On occasions, we are aware that if we *had* a particular ability we would not need to refer the patient for an opinion or for a procedure. With the PUNs & DENs approach, we learn to *record* these experiences and use them to identify and prioritise what we need to learn.

The technique has some advantages and disadvantages.

Advantages

Being based on the bedrock of general practice, the consultation, greatly increases the validity of the technique as the areas of educational need that it identifies are derived first-hand from what we do with our patients. It is simple to use, immediate and relatively unobtrusive and can be used in *any* clinical encounter, i.e. telephone consultations as well as those we conduct face to face.

The use of this method doesn't generate much anxiety as it is usually a form of self-assessment. Additionally, the act of thinking about PUNs makes us more patient-centred and this in itself may improve our consulting skills. Recording PUNs also makes it more likely that we will act on them.

Compared with other forms of assessment, many of the DENs demonstrated can be quickly addressed, for example by looking something up in a book or finding out about where to refer a patient, and therefore this approach can rapidly produce benefit for our patients and for ourselves.

Disadvantages

It is *subjective* and is dependent on our skill at disclosing a patient's need, our ability to recognise a need once disclosed and our honesty in admitting that the need was unmet. Because each consultation may disclose PUNs & DENs, many educational needs may quickly be uncovered and this *may prove de-motivating* if we find it difficult to sort the wheat from the chaff. The record made is a negative one, in that it is an account of all the things that we did not do and what this might indicate about our deficiencies. To compensate for this we need to learn to *recognise our strengths* at the same time as recording our PUNs & DENs.

The process of recording PUNs needs to take place either after each consultation or at the end of surgery while the events are clear in our minds, and this will therefore make our surgeries last longer.

How can individuals use them?

Using PUNs & DENs is a simple approach with obvious charm, but care needs to be taken that it does not become simplistic. There is the danger that we might regard all unmet needs as necessarily indicating an educational need. This is certainly not the case, and indeed the more skilled we become at consulting, the more we encourage patients to open up and to disclose their needs. We therefore have to consider to what extent these 'patient needs' should be addressed, if at all, by ourselves.

Because they are usually restricted to the consultation and therefore do not formally take into account the other areas of our work, PUNs & DENs should not be relied on alone but should be part of a broader strategy to identify our learning needs. Such an approach could look at our referral patterns and our prescribing and service delivery, perhaps by comparing these with colleagues within the practice or the PCG/LHG.

PUNs & DENs offer a snapshot view of our performance that looks quite widely but relatively superficially at what we do, and this can be complemented by forms of assessment such as audit, which look more deeply and over a longer timescale at our work.

The technique develops our self-awareness but may ignore the perspectives of others, such as our fellow practitioners and indeed our patients, unless we seek to obtain them. How close, I wonder, is the correlation between what *we* perceive to be a patient need and what the patient himself thinks?

How do we use PUNs & DENs in our consultations?

Identifying PUNs

Despite the limitations mentioned above, the approach is both powerful and useful, so how could we go about identifying PUNs & DENs? The following represents one method.

We need to adopt an appropriate mind-set. Although we are likely to uncover many unmet needs, this does not mean that we are bad or negligent doctors – just honest ones!

Especially in the early days, we should ensure that our experience of this technique is a positive one. As well as PUNs, there will be many PAMs – *Patients Actually Met* needs (apologies to Dr Eve) and we should recognise these and pat ourselves on the back for them.

The approach requires us to think about the content of the consultation as soon after the interaction as possible. In particular, we should think about the presenting complaint, any hidden agenda, and the patient's ideas, concerns and expectations regarding the consultation. We should consider to what extent we determined any or all of these by, for example, asking ourselves whether we enquired of the patient what *their* thoughts were?

Next, we need to consider which management options were arrived at and whether we shared these with the patient. If we did, the patient may have voiced a preference for the problem to be managed in a particular way and we should consider whether this wish was respected, and if not, for what reasons. Might it have been that we lacked the ability to implement a particular option? If so an educational need may have been demonstrated.

Sometimes we are only aware that a PUN might have been present because the outcome of the consultation was unsatisfactory, with one or both parties feeling dissatisfied. Dissatisfaction is a sign that a need has not been met and that there are lessons to be learned by reflecting on this.

PUNs may not be obvious to us and may need to be arrived at by inference. We can improve our 'hit rate' at detecting PUNs through practice and by watching video consultations of ourselves and of others. In particular, video analysis allows us to witness the non-verbal cues which can signify so much, but which are frequently overlooked. So often it is these cues that show us how our patients *really* feel. In addition, we can be critical in a safe environment about the techniques we use to establish rapport, and can decide how to modify our use of verbal and non-verbal language in order to discover what our patients' needs are.

Making a record

Having identified the PUNs, we should make a note of them as soon after the consultation as possible, although it may take a few days before we can decide what the corresponding DENs are.

An example of a completed PUNs and DENs analysis sheet is shown in Table 6.1 at the end of this chapter – we now look at each section of this sheet and consider how it should be completed.

Consultation

Make a one-line note to remind ourselves of the consultation and its circumstances (remember we may not be acting on this information for a little while).

PUNs

On reflection, which PUNs did we identify? We need to be as precise as possible, framing PUNs in such a way as to make it easier to translate them into specific educational needs. It is preferable, especially when new to this technique, not to overlook any PUNs, for reasons explained below.

Why were the needs unmet?

Make a note of our thoughts. Remember that this is a record made by ourselves for ourselves, so we can afford to be honest. Such honesty is important because it helps us to decide why certain PUNs occurred and therefore how significant they are.

It is helpful to think about the reasons in terms of deficiencies in *knowledge*, *skills*, *attitudes* and *resources*. For example, suppose that a 68-year-old woman complains incidentally of occasional dizziness and paraesthesae for the past four months. We may not meet her need for advice about this condition because of a lack of:

- *knowledge* of the differential diagnosis
- *skill* in performing a neurological examination
- an appropriate *attitude*, perhaps believing her symptoms to be trivial, or
- *resources*, in that we are running late and haven't the time to investigate further.

DENs

Now look at the PUNs and the reasons for them, as we should be able to categorise our deficiency in the manner shown above by using this information. Resources were mentioned because it is important to know that sometimes needs are unmet for reasons that cannot be remedied through the further education of the doctor.

Next, we should write down how the deficiency we have identified could be corrected. We needn't worry at this stage about *precisely* how it could be done as that is the purpose of our personal development plan, but instead we should state our learning needs in general terms. For example, for the patient with dizziness we may write 'I feel ignorant about this topic and I need to read about the diagnosis and management of dizziness in the elderly'. Some deficiencies are easy to identify but difficult to correct, so that in the example given we may have regarded the patient's dizziness as being trivial and then have written, 'My problem is to do with my attitude towards this patient. I need to find out *why* I regard her complaints as trivial'.

It was mentioned that we should not *ignore* those unmet needs that we disclose. This is because over a series of consultations we may find that the same, seemingly unimportant, unmet needs keep recurring. Suppose that we discovered over the course of time that we failed to examine elderly women with symptoms of pruritis vulvae. We might then ask ourselves why the patient's 'need' to have a diagnosis properly established remained unmet. Could it be that we felt uncomfortable about gynaecological examinations in the elderly, or were unsure what leukoplakia might look like?

In the psychological domain, we might note that a patient seemed dissatisfied with the outcome of the consultation and record this as a PUN. After a series of consultations in which the same PUN recurred we might find that the common denominator was a presenting symptom of tiredness and this might lead us to consider whether we were failing to consider depression in patients presenting with this symptom.

Action

Having decided on our educational need, the next task is to determine how to address it. For this, we need to write down the initial step that we intend to take. The purpose of the 'action' box is not to define exactly how the educational need will be met but rather to act as a catalyst to ensure that progress occurs. To this end it is important that our first step is feasible given the resources that are available, and that the timescale is one which we know can be achieved. Once these targets have been set, achieving them forms part of our PDP, for which we need to think about how we can demonstrate to ourselves and to others that our needs have been met and that our behaviour has changed.

At its most basic level, this evidence may come from observing our future PUNs & DENs – do they confirm that the same unmet needs do not keep recurring? More sophisticated evidence of learning may be in the form of teaching others, writing a guideline or protocol, or conducting an audit. This should not put us off, however, as committing ourselves to do no more than just *think* about what we have learned is a good place to start.

Inviting others to contribute to our PUNs & DENs exercise is not mandatory, but can greatly increase its value. Asking a colleague to consider our activity in consultation by looking at our PUNs & DENs analysis sheet and hearing our thoughts, or perhaps by watching a video of our consultations, gives us the opportunity to gain a different perspective and hopefully a greater insight into our skills. Such colleagues may also be able to help with regard to how our educational needs could be met. Most doctors regard such an invitation to contribute as a privilege, and links established in this way can improve relationships greatly. Who knows, you may be asked to return the favour!

How could the practice team use PUNs & DENs?

Determining PUNs & DENs not only helps the individual to recognise their strengths and weaknesses, but also, if the information is shared, helps a team to build up a profile of the range of knowledge and skills possessed by its members. Using such a profile, priorities for education can be set because when an educational deficiency is common to several members of the team, then a *Team Educational Need* (a *TEN* rather than a *DEN*) has been demonstrated.

The PUNs & DENs of the team could also be determined by conducting other forms of assessment. For example, an audit of clinical care or of patient complaints may highlight differences between partners from which PUNs could be inferred and DENs derived.

When individuals undertake their own PUNs & DENs exercise, they obtain comments from their colleagues only by inviting them. If the *team* uses the technique in the way described it is vital that the individuals assessed are handled sensitively both with regard to how deficiencies are exposed and how these might be remedied. One approach is to use the method described for team-based feedback in Chapter 7, on significant event analysis.

Just as doctors have to make arrangements to attend to their DENs, if a TEN is present it may be worthwhile and cost-effective to arrange for group tuition. 'Educational resources' usually means people with particular knowledge, *experience* or skills, and such resources could be shared on a reciprocal arrangement between teams.

I've highlighted the word 'experience', because this is something we *all* acquire from the earliest stages of our careers. People who have experience are often the best teachers, as they know immediately what the difficulties are and how best to overcome them. As housemen, doctors are used to the maxim 'see one, do one, teach one' and often consider that they learn much more from practitioners than they do from reading the books. Therefore, can I seed this thought in your minds: don't our experiences as GPs make us *all* potential teachers?

Summary

As we can see, the PUNs & DENs approach is an extremely practical one. In our own ways, we use it frequently but never glorify it with a title! So much then for the theory – if the approach interests you, you can obtain the analysis sheets, or logbooks as they are called, from the address given opposite. Try it for yourself.

Obtaining logbooks

Logbooks to record your discoveries, including instruction and examples, can be obtained for £3.00 + p&p from: Dr Richard Eve, Lime Tree, Mount Street, Bishops Lydeard, Taunton TA4 3LH. *Tel*: 01823 432089; *Fax*: 01823 326755; *e-mail*: eve97@msn.com

Table 6.1: PUNs & DENs: analysis sheet

No.	Consultation details	PUNs identified	Why were the needs unmet?	DENs – what deficiencies have you identified?	Action
1	42-year-old woman with a painful heel treated with NSAIDs by my partner for two weeks. Minimal improvement	Diagnosed plantar fasciitis – patient needed a steroid injection which she didn't get	I've never done one before and didn't feel I had the skill	I need to learn how to give this soft-tissue injection	One of my partners does a minor surgery clinic. I will sit in with her, learn how to give the injection and do my first one under her supervision
2	The parents of a 15-year-old boy – very worried because his behaviour has recently become uncontrollable	They asked how they would know whether their son was taking drugs. I was evasive	I wasn't sure of my facts or where to direct them for further advice	I need to find out more specifically about the signs of drug abuse in teenagers. I also need to increase my awareness of local resources which could help these kids and their parents	Contact the substance abuse clinic for advice about resources and appropriate reading for myself. Contact the health authority regarding useful leaflets (we could use some in our waiting room)

Table 6.1: PUNs & DENs: analysis sheet *continued*

No.	Consultation details	PUNs identified	Why were the needs unmet?	DENs – what deficiencies have you identified?	Action
3	A very sensible 72-year-old man, hypertensive with reasonably controlled BP, asked me if he should be taking aspirin for his health. There were no contraindications and he had no further risk factors. Turns out he's buying it anyway	A very good question! Unfortunately I didn't have the answer	I'm pretty confident about the use of aspirin in secondary prevention of coronary heart disease and stroke, but I'm hazy (and to be honest, confused) about its use in primary prevention	I need to find out about the use of aspirin in hypertensive patients with no other risk factors. I also need to think about the implications for the practice of recommending this strategy	Start by ringing the cardiology registrar. I'll also bring it up at the next team meeting – I wonder what my partners are recommending? I really ought to do a literature search but I'm not sure how (another DEN!)

7 Significant event analysis (SEA)

Key points

- Significant events in our professional lives can be examples of when things go significantly right as well as significantly wrong.
- They can be analysed through personal reflection or in larger groups.
- Discussing them with the practice team allows whole-patient care across the team to be assessed.
- The outcomes of SEA include celebration or the recognition of good practice, as well as the demonstration of a need for audit or for an immediate change in behaviour.
- Significant events can be used systematically to study particular areas of our service.
- These areas may be organisational as well as clinical.
- There are some ground rules for the way in which significant events are discussed, which maximise the benefits of the process.
- Keeping records allows the team to learn, and individuals to use the experience in forming their PDPs.

What is SEA?

Of the many events that happen to and around us in practice life, significant events are those which make an impact on the mind (and the heart). They can be examples of when things go significantly *right* as well as significantly wrong and can be clinical or non-clinical events, involving anyone from one person to the entire team. Because *we* regard them as significant, they are powerful motivators for change, and this can be harnessed through the process of significant event analysis (SEA).

SEA is the mechanism by which we look at noteworthy events in our practice lives with the purpose of learning from and celebrating good practice as well as improving suboptimal practice. The great benefit which people derive from SEA is out of proportion to the effort it requires.

What's in a name?

SEA seems to go by various names: significant event audit, critical event audit or analysis, significant event review and so on.

I have chosen the term 'significant event' because the term 'critical' implies incidents which are negative in their consequences, which as we have said, is not always so. I have used 'analysis' because this term is broad-ranging and does not commit us to undertaking an audit cycle.

How can SEA help us?

Let us illustrate this with an example: suppose that we visit a 53-year-old man with a history of hypertension and angina who has a prolonged episode of chest pain. Tragically, he dies at home of an MI before the ambulance arrives.

We could look at this incident to determine whether there are any lessons to be learned, by asking ourselves the following questions:

- What went well?
- What went badly?
- How could I improve?

The answer to the last question might identify a learning need that we could use in our PDP.

This simple analysis could be done quickly, perhaps in discussion with a colleague and would involve a minimum of paperwork. However, we could go one step further and discuss the same incident with our teams, thus using the full potential of SEA to assess the quality of service delivered by *all* those involved in the patient's care. The sort of questions that might be asked of different team members and services are illustrated below.

Doctors

- This patient had a history of CHD. Was he receiving secondary prevention? Was he checked for other risk factors? How well was his hypertension managed? Was his BP checked regularly and treated in accordance with the British Hypertension Society guidelines?
- How well was his angina controlled? Were there any warning symptoms in the recent past? Had his vascular status been assessed at the hospital?
- How quickly was the doctor in attendance following the visit request?
- What acute therapy was given?
- Did the doctor carry a defibrillator, and if so, did he know how to use it?

Practice nurses

- What responsibility did they have in the patient's management?
- Were the chronic disease management protocols upheld?
- Was lifestyle advice given and smoking status recorded?
- Was compliance with treatment checked?
- Was non-attendance followed up?

Receptionists

- How was the request for the visit handled?
- Was an urgent visit requested – if not, should it have been prioritised anyway?

- Were any recent requests for appointments deferred, and if so was this appropriate?

Ambulance services

- Was there any difficulty contacting the service?
- Was the response time adequate?

This list is not intended to be exhaustive, but it gives an idea of the range of disciplines involved in a single significant event and of the range of questions that we might choose to ask. It also demonstrates our interdependence and the fact that good-quality care requires competence at *all* levels.

Performing a SEA using this incident could lead to one of four outcomes.

The need for immediate change

Suppose that it came to light that the patient had come to surgery the day before, complained to the receptionist of worsening angina, but had not been given an immediate appointment. This incident could be used to educate receptionists to respond appropriately to alarm symptoms of this type.

Demonstration of the need for an audit

Perhaps this patient's BP had not been well-controlled. An audit of hypertension management would reveal whether this was an isolated case or whether standards needed to be improved more generally. An audit might also show where the deficiency lay – whether it was due to management by particular doctors, particular nurses or perhaps due to a problem with the clinic protocol, for example.

Recognition of good practice

Whereby all that could have been done, had been done. The team could feel justifiably proud of attaining high standards in the knowledge that although this tragedy happened, they could not have prevented it.

Celebration

Although this sounds incongruous, celebration may be justified where exemplary care is seen. For example, the GP might have appropriately administered thrombolytic drugs, where this was not yet common practice in the area. In other circumstances, where exemplary practice *succeeds* in averting a patient from harm, the cause for celebration is easier to accept.

Because SEA looks at the performance of several people, it is possible that more than one outcome will be seen. Thus some individuals or groups will see their actions vindicated or praised, while others will acknowledge that there is work to be done. The way in which feedback is given is therefore highly important if the team as a whole is not to be divided.

As we can see, even if we thought that the significant event did not involve us directly, attending a SEA meeting may make us look at our actions and thereby bring to light learning needs of which we were previously unaware.

What types of significant event are there?

We define events as being significant because they are thought to be important in our professional lives or the life of the practice, or because they may offer some insight into the standards of care that the practice provides. Most people start with events that are dramatic by virtue of their nature or consequences, and use these to learn from.

Examples of these include:

- a sudden unexpected death in the community
- a patient who behaves violently in the waiting room
- the theft of a prescription pad.

We can learn from these as they arise, in which case the areas of personal and practice activity that we end up examining are a matter of chance. Another approach is to keep a record of significant events when they occur, and categorise them according to the area of activity into which they fall. We can then audit our service systematically by choosing an area and analysing the event associated with it.

Examples of these areas are:

- clinical: preventive, acute and chronic
- organisational.

Let us now consider these areas in more detail with some examples of significant events in each and how they could be used.

Clinical: preventive care

Unplanned pregnancy

The UK has the highest rate of unwanted teenage pregnancies in Western Europe. When such an event occurs in our practice, we could use it as an opportunity to examine the team approach to sexual health:

- How accessible are the family planning clinics?
- How approachable is the service to teenagers, especially the under-16s.
- What is the age distribution of patients seen in clinic?
- What about emergency contraception: what advice are patients receiving, and does the practice offer an urgent appointment when the 'morning-after pill' is requested?

Other examples of significant events in preventive care: *positive cervical smear, congenital dislocation of the hip, orchidopexy.*

If these events were found to be rare, then SEA would have the effect of showing that high standards of preventive care are being achieved.

Clinical: acute care

Serious diagnosis

A serious diagnosis, such as a new cancer diagnosis, prompts us to review the patient records and ask:

- When was the condition first diagnosed?
- When did the patient first present with symptoms which in retrospect might have been attributable to the illness?

- Could we reasonably say that the condition should have been suspected at an earlier stage?
- When was the patient referred – should this have been done sooner?
- How quickly was the patient seen after referral – was this acceptable?

It may well be that the patient was examined at the first presentation, referred and seen urgently and hence no delay occurred.

Missed diagnosis

These are diagnoses which we could or should have made, but failed to do. For example, the young man with recurrent night sweats may turn out not to have flu but a lymphoma, and the girl who isn't concentrating at school may not have a behaviour problem but epilepsy.

These diagnoses usually come to light when another healthcare professional is involved and this raises two additional points. First, while we are ready to involve another professional (usually a consultant and therefore not a peer) when we are having clinical difficulties, we are less willing to see our deficiencies uncovered by our practice colleagues or indeed by our patients.

Being 'exposed' in this way may amount to no more than seeing an entry in the clinical records when another partner has been involved in the patient's care, some friendly feedback from a colleague over a cup of coffee, or a patient prompting us with an article from a newspaper about a condition which seems to fit their symptoms. These incidents are opportunities for education and improvement even though they may initially feel like unwelcome criticism.

Second, it is important that colleagues who uncover such missed diagnoses take the opportunity to let the relevant parties learn from the incident while exercising sensitivity over the manner and forum in which they do so.

Other examples of significant events in acute care: *sudden infant death syndrome, attempted suicide, cerebrovascular accident (CVA).*

Clinical: chronic care

Child admitted with asthma

Thankfully, asthma deaths are now rare. However, asthma admissions remain relatively common, and we could use such an event to audit the child's asthma management by asking such questions as:

- Was the child taking part in a disease management programme?
- How often was he attending the asthma clinic?
- Were symptom enquiries and peak flow measurements routinely being performed in the clinic?
- What was the inhaler technique like?
- Was prophylaxis being used at the optimal level.
- Do we know if the parents smoke?
- Did he have, or need, a written management plan?
- Did the parents know when to call for advice?

Other examples of significant events in chronic care: *Status epilepticus, below-knee amputation in a known diabetic, CVA in a known hypertensive.*

Organisational

This heading covers a multitude of sins – and successes! Significant events can occur in many non-clinical domains of practice life so let us look at some examples in these areas.

Service delivery

An important route by which shortcomings in the delivery of care can be highlighted is the patient complaint. We have always taken complaints seriously, and nowadays there is a contractual duty to deal with them in a professional manner. However, this duty does not require us to discuss the lessons learned but merely to report that the process has been observed and that the outcome has, or has not, been successful.

Patient complaints can highlight aspects of the quality, range and accessibility of both our clinical and non-clinical services. As partners in healthcare, patients are

increasingly being encouraged to contribute and their suggestions for improvement, as well as their positive feedback regarding our services, could be used as
significant events from which to learn.

Practice management

- *Problems with protocols*: as an illustration, consider the situation in which there
  is a delay in responding to an emergency visit request either because there is no
  protocol regarding how such requests are passed on, or because the protocol
  that exists is inadequate. Such a protocol may not stipulate, for example, who is
  responsible for passing the request on, what to do if the doctor is not
  contactable or under what circumstances an emergency ambulance can be
  ordered by the receptionist.

- *Staff management*: significant events may arise as a result of mistakes,
  sometimes brought to light through the feedback or complaints of patients or
  through the routine supervision of practice activity. This may highlight training
  issues, but the areas of performance review, employment law and disciplinary
  action may also need to be considered. Staff may themselves be upset by the
  behaviour of the patients or, dare I say it, the doctors, thus creating other issues
  which need to be addressed.

We should not forget that there are numerous examples relating to staff, in which
difficult situations are managed particularly well by individuals or groups. These
significant events should be used as opportunities to demonstrate to them that
their efforts are noticed and appreciated by their colleagues, a token which is often
valued more by individuals than the financial rewards of their work.

- *Financial management*: significant events may include payment claims that are
  missed through poor book-keeping, thus reducing the opportunity to
  maximise practice income. For example, the practice may fail to achieve the full
  minor surgery payment because the doctors were not informed how many
  more procedures they should have notified by the end of the quarter year.

- *Estate management*: by which I mean attending to the practice building and
  contents. Water damage may force us to attend to the upkeep of the surgery
  roof; and a burglary might prompt a review of the security arrangements and
  insurance cover.

Less dramatic events can be studied in order to prevent future disasters. For example, an electric heater left on overnight might just be considered to be a disciplinary matter. However, used as a significant event, it could encourage the practice to review the fire regulations for public buildings, to invite the local fire officer to inspect the building and make recommendations, and to ensure that the practice staff engage in a periodic fire drill.

How can we conduct a SEA?

The key point here is that SEA should be felt to be a positive experience by those involved in it. The fact that we are engaging in the process at all is itself commendable and this should be recognised.

Who is going to be involved, when and where?

Most significant events involve several people in the team and it is usually appropriate for those involved in the event to discuss and learn from the experience together. Doctors and nurses are used to putting time aside for what they regard as professional development. However, SEA may well require the attendance of employees (receptionists, practice manager, computer operator, etc.) and protected time will have to be arranged. Note that the implication is that doctors or nurses make the decision as to which events will be discussed and in what sort of forum. As practice teams develop it is hoped that other members, such as employees, will be similarly empowered.

How soon after a significant event should it be analysed? This depends largely on the event, with those that may indicate a serious shortcoming requiring immediate attention. With other events it is useful to have time to reflect on matters before formally conducting a SEA, but the length of time should not be too great otherwise momentum will be lost and details forgotten. Hence details of a significant event should be recorded as soon as we become aware that one has taken place.

Getting into the habit of routinely conducting SEA means that any anxiety associated with the process is reduced and the experience becomes more influential in shaping our future behaviour.

SEA is not just an uncovering of facts and the formulation of action points – there are sometimes strong feelings involved and it is important that the group is not interrupted from without or within (mobile phones and bleeps). You may wish to consider which environment is the most conducive. Meetings outside the workplace are more likely to encourage people to open up, but may be less convenient and less focused on problem solving.

What are the ground rules?

SEA requires participants to be honest with each other, and those involved must feel that they have entered into the process willingly and are both prepared to play an active part and to learn from the experience. Confidentiality should not be assumed and some clear guidelines should be established as to what could be discussed outside the group.

So how do you get it right? One approach is to ask others who have conducted SEA to advise you, or even help you by facilitating a meeting. In return, as your experience develops you may be able to offer a similar service to others. Just as doctors can mentor each other, so practices can provide co-facilitation.

Even if a facilitator is not used, meetings of more than four people generally need a chairperson to make sure that all have a chance to contribute, that conflict does not occur and that appropriate records are kept. These records are usually a note of the significant event itself, what went well, what went badly and as a result of discussion, the recommendations being made for improvement.

Let us now consider the key stages in conducting a SEA. The process is described for a significant event with negative connotations, only because these are the types most often discussed. When positive events are analysed not all the points made below will be relevant.

Why has this significant event been chosen?

It is useful to establish why this event is significant and to determine what those involved wish to achieve by analysing it. Sometimes the process starts with an individual who feels unhappy, perhaps guilty about an event and wishes to explore it further, in which case the purpose of SEA is partly to address that need. At other times personal feelings may not be involved but there may be an issue of practice performance that needs to be addressed collectively.

What are the facts of the case?

To save time it is useful to circulate the factual material relating to the event, such as the date and time, nature of the event, the circumstances and people involved, prior to the meeting. Those principally involved will need to have done some background work, perhaps by reviewing the patient records or establishing the sequence of events. In addition, they should be prepared to talk about how the event was managed and whether there are, or might be, longer-term consequences.

For many significant events the only 'props' needed for SEA are the patient records, but any relevant material should be brought to the meeting.

What issues are raised?

Having clarified the facts the next stage is to decide what issues are raised by the event. We will want to consider each of these issues in turn in order to decide if any action is needed. To illustrate this, consider the example given earlier regarding the 53-year-old man who dies at home following an MI. We could list some of the issues as follows:

- emergency clinical care – drugs and equipment, etc.
- communication – dealing with an emergency request, doctor and ambulance response times.
- preventive care – clinical management, follow-up, etc.

What went well?

With these issues in mind, those involved should discuss the areas relating to the event that they feel generally positive about. This helps to put the event into perspective and once they have spoken, others in the group should be encouraged to voice their observations of the examples of good practice that the event demonstrates – and there are always some.

What went badly and how could we improve?

What was it exactly that went wrong? It is important to be specific, as this helps to differentiate significant lapses in performance from the 'feel bad' surrounding the event. To achieve this, the key members should be given time to go through the following stages:

1 Talk about what went wrong.
2 Discuss their feelings with respect to the event itself.
3 Describe how they might have done things differently.
4 Discuss what they might have needed in order to do things differently in terms of knowledge, skills and resources. This step highlights areas for possible action.
5 *Invite* others in the group to make their comments. I emphasise the word invite because if the key members are encouraged to retain control at this point, their feelings of vulnerability will be reduced and they will be more likely to take note of the comments made.

Those invited, and it may be a general invitation to the whole group, could proceed along the following lines:

1 Select the major shortcoming that they perceive. Because the purpose of feedback is to improve future performance, this shortcoming should preferably be one that is amenable to improvement.
2 Point out any alternative strategy that may have prevented the problem or allowed it to have been more effectively managed.
3 Highlight any skills or resources that may be needed by the person concerned to enact the suggested strategy in future.
4 Make their final comments positive ones, perhaps by reiterating what the colleague has done well, and thus encouraging him to improve. This step is important because people particularly tend to remember the last thing that someone has said to them.

This stage of SEA would need modification if we were talking with groups of people who were jointly involved in a significant event. Personal sensibilities may not be such an issue and time constraints may not allow *individuals* to go through all the steps listed above.

Which improvements are feasible?

Having heard the deliberations of the group it is useful to summarise the key points of what went wrong and the suggestions made for improvement. We now have to decide on the appropriate action by determining which of the suggestions made are feasible, and which of these should be prioritised. This approach is a practical one which recognises that not all the factors that contribute to a problem can be remedied.

What action should be taken?

Action may involve formulating a plan based on one or more steps from the following scheme:

1 Decide which improvements are to be prioritised.

2 Determine which new skills or resources are needed to meet these requirements.

3 Plan for these needs to be met.

4 Decide on a timescale over which the improvements are to be made.

5 Consider whether and how to widen the educational benefit gained by the participants in this SEA, bearing in mind confidentiality issues and the need to anonymise information.

6 Consider how the success of this action plan could be determined. Are there elements in the suggested improvements that can be measured and therefore audited?

What records should we keep?

Overwhelmed as we are by paperwork it is tempting to avoid the written word when we can. With SEA this is almost always a mistake. Making a record offers the following advantages:

• Writing down the circumstances of the event helps to clarify the facts and avoid misunderstanding.

• A record can be made of the analysis itself and what action was taken as a result. This can serve as a useful summary of why things went wrong and the lessons that were learned. In the future, faced with similar circumstances this information could prove valuable.

- Appropriate details from the record can be shared in a suitable form with a wider audience, e.g. specific details can be fed back to a patient who made a complaint or anonymised information can be given to colleagues outside the practice who wish to learn from our experience.
- The process of SEA is a form of adult learning. Making a record of the deliberations could allow the time spent to be accredited as part of our PDP.

Significant event examples and analysis sheets

The practice could decide what the record should contain, but I have provided two examples of the sort of record that could be made.

The first is an abbreviated record such as could be kept to note the main outcomes of a SEA meeting. The second is a more detailed record which individuals could complete for their PDPs. This record uses questions which are split into two sections – the first uses questions that encourage reflection on the significant event, and the second questions that help us to plan our learning.

Examples demonstrating how the sheets could be completed are given, followed by blank sheets for your own use.

Summary

Most GPs can't help talking about their work. It fascinates us, and we are often keen to share anything that is out of the ordinary with our colleagues. We also seem to instinctively realise that significant events are a rich vein from which to extract our learning. Capturing and making constructive use of this fascination with the unusual is the essence of significant event analysis, and of all the techniques discussed in this book, it is the one which even in the most rudimentary form, I would urge you to make use of.

Further information

Pringle M, Bradley C, Carmichael C, Wallis H and Moore A (1995) *Significant Event Auditing.* Occasional Paper No. 70. Royal College of General Practitioners, London.

This paper explains the principles of SEA in more detail, particularly the way in which SEA is used by practices to audit their care.

Significant event: Saturday morning emergency surgery – patient behaved in an aggressive manner towards the receptionist

Issues arising from discussion	• Staff safety • Security of premises • Panic buttons • Removal of patients from the list
Positive points	• Patient was calmed down by receptionist • Doctor was alerted without inflaming the situation • Patient was recognised as being ill (schizophrenic) and not subsequently removed from the list
Concerns	• Potential for harm: receptionist was on her own, waiting room was otherwise empty • Patient was able to lean across into reception area • There was no panic button to call for help
Suggestions	• Ensure that two receptionists are always working together • Redesign reception counter • Install panic buttons • Consider staff training • Ask the advice of the local police
Action	• Training session organised for the team regarding how to manage potentially violent patients • Arrange quotes for new fixtures • Apply for grant for this equipment • Ensure that phones in the reception area have a direct dial to the police station

Significant event

Issues arising from discussion

Positive points

Concerns

Suggestions

Action

Significant event analysis sheet – *Reflection*

1 Description of the event
- Missed diagnosis of cholesteatoma
- A 32-year-old woman who had a 13-year history of right-sided otalgia was diagnosed by a locum doctor, having been treated numerous times for a discharging right ear by various doctors in the practice, most recently by myself

2 Issues raised by the event
- The diagnosis was missed: was the possibility of cholesteatoma not considered, perhaps through ignorance?
- Record keeping: there were numerous attendances – why was the pattern not recognised?
- Safety netting: what follow-up was arranged after each attendance?

3 What went well
- The patient was seen and examined each time that she attended with an ear problem
- Adequate notes were kept, the patient was (eventually) correctly diagnosed and managed
- The situation was discussed with her, and she did not wish to make a complaint

4 What didn't go well
- The diagnosis could have been made earlier, and wasn't
- Previous attendances over several years were not recognised
- The patient was either not asked to return following treatment for a discharging ear, or failed to return when requested

5 How I might have done things differently
- Taken more time to look back over the medical records
- Asked the patient to return following treatment
- Arranged to recall the patient when she failed to attend
- Had a higher index of suspicion in a patient with a chronic ear infection

Significant event analysis sheet – *Reflection*

1 Description of the event

2 Issues raised by the event

3 What went well

4 What didn't go well

5 How I might have done things differently

Significant event analysis sheet – *Action*

6 Areas of feasible improvement

- Improve recognition of recurrent problems in the patient records
- Improve safety netting
- Improve management of chronic ear infections

7 Educational needs identified

- Learn how to identify active clinical problems using the computer
- Read about the management of chronic ear infections
- Learn to recognise cholesteatomata, and the risk factors for them

8 Which needs I will address and in what order

- All the above
- I will attend to clinical areas first

9 How I intend to meet those needs

- Read the relevant chapters in an ENT textbook
- Attend an ENT clinic

10 How I will be able to demonstrate improvement

- Over a six-month period, I will use the computer to code patients with chronic ear infections whom I manage
- Using this information I will conduct an audit of the case management of these patients

Significant event analysis sheet – *Action*

6 Areas of feasible improvement

7 Educational needs identified

8 Which needs I will address and in what order

9 How I intend to meet those needs

10 How I will be able to demonstrate improvement

8 Clinical audit

Introduction

What is clinical audit?

How could it help me?

Who does the audit?

How do I conduct an audit?

Who can help me?

Summary

Key points

- Audit is the method by which we look systematically and critically at our work with the objective of improving patient care.

- It can help us to identify deficiencies, encourage us to change and reduce the errors that we might make. It can also demonstrate good standards of care.

- Audits can be performed by ourselves, in association with our colleagues or by external assessors.

- Audit is not about 'naming and shaming', but about encouraging improvements in performance within a supportive environment.

- The audit process involves setting standards and measuring our performance against these.

- Making changes in order to improve our performance and then repeating the audit is the mechanism by which we complete the audit cycle.

- Various agencies can advise as to how to engage in audit, and audit protocols are readily available.

Introduction

From a once-esoteric activity, audit is becoming more commonplace, spurred on by Primary Care Audit Groups and the process of summative assessment, which requires GP registrars to successfully complete an audit project before being certified for independent practice. Audit is often used for practice management and practices that are well-run, profitable and deliver high-quality care almost always incorporate audit as part of their routine activity.

Here, we are concerned with how audit can help us from an educational viewpoint and our focus will be on clinical audit activity. We will look first at the benefits of engaging in clinical audit and then go on to consider in more detail how it can be undertaken, some of the difficulties involved and how we can ensure that our efforts bear fruit.

What is clinical audit?

Put simply, clinical audit is the method by which health professionals look systematically and critically at their work with the purpose of enhancing the health and quality of life of their patients.

Previously, clinical audit usually involved a group of doctors getting together to analyse and learn from their work. In more recent times it is becoming recognised that the delivery of healthcare involves many disciplines within primary care and as a result, audit activity is becoming a joint venture within practices, and indeed, between practices. One insight from this multidisciplinary approach, is the extent to which one team member is dependent on the quality of work of the others – in other words, the end product is only as good as its weakest link.

To those who have not taken part in audit before, there are some common misconceptions which serve to give it a forbidding image. Here are some things that audit is *not*:

- It is *not* 'research'. In research we are unclear what 'best practice' represents and the purpose of our activity is to try and find out. In audit, we not only know what we need to do but we are able to state how well we should be able to do it.

- An audit is *not just number crunching*. In the past, GPs have been required to provide facts and figures and to engage in so-called audit activity that in reality was little more than data collection. In clinical audit, we have ownership of the process and we decide what data to collect on the basis of what *we* are trying to study and how best to use that data to improve our standards. Done in this way, audit is far from a sterile activity.
- Audit is *not about 'naming and shaming'* – it allows those whose work is being analysed to recognise where their weaknesses lie but this is very much within an environment of support. The best audits come to nothing if it is not recognised that people need to be acknowledged for their strengths and encouraged and supported to make the improvements that audit recommends.

How could it help me?

Some of the reasons why audit is worth engaging in are listed below.

Identifying deficiencies

Clinical audit can help to identify some of our strengths and weaknesses. Often, the subject of the audit is decided on by a group of people on the basis of the interests of the practice. We may not know at the outset whether we have an area of personal deficiency and although the outcome of the audit may sometimes confirm our worst fears, it may also show that our best hopes regarding our performance are justified.

Sometimes we may choose to undertake an audit for personal reasons, perhaps because we suspect that we have a problem area and wish to discover whether this is the case, and if so to what extent. Audit not only allows us to identify an area that needs our attention but also provides the means, through the comparison of our performance against standards which we set, of measuring the improvements that we try to make.

Encouraging change

Many changes that GPs are subjected to are externally imposed, but with audit we have the opportunity to decide where the priorities lie within our practices, and hence where change is needed.

Audit requires us to look objectively at the topic being considered and learn more about it before deciding on the criteria and standards. This means that when, as a group, we try to define 'best practice', we challenge the *evidence* rather than each other's opinion. Later, when the audit is performed, the data allow comparisons to be made objectively.

Hence, by increasing ownership, establishing an evidence-base and depersonalising the arguments by using data rather than impressions to make comparisons, audit encourages change.

Reduces errors

We have touched on one form of 'error' which audit may highlight, namely that we are not treating our patients in line with currently accepted 'best practice'. This type of error can be corrected through learning.

Quite often though, we know what we should be doing but not whether we are actually doing it. Audit is a powerful tool for showing us how diligent (or otherwise) we are at putting into practice what we have learned. In addition, when changes are made and new standards or protocols are agreed, audit is the mechanism by which team members can prove to themselves and to others that protocols are being implemented.

We have said that audit is not about apportioning blame. To succeed in producing change, audit doesn't need to publicly ascribe blame to the individual, but *does* need to allow those involved to make comparisons. GPs often compare themselves with their peers and don't like to be seen as 'below average', and this proves to be a powerful motivator for self-improvement. This factor should be borne in mind when audit results are discussed.

What sort of audit can expose potential clinical errors? Let us take as an example an audit of the management of epilepsy and ask ourselves for what percentage of our epileptic patients we could claim that:

- patients coded with epilepsy have been correctly diagnosed
- known epileptics have a disease coding
- known epileptics on anti-convulsant therapy have their medication reviewed at least once a year
- at the review, epileptics are questioned about side effects, driving status and contraception (where appropriate).

Even simple audits like this are likely to uncover significant gaps in care, some of which may have medico-legal implications. Hence, reducing error through audit is an important way of preventing harm to the patient and of reducing the risk to ourselves.

Demonstrating good care

We might believe that our practice delivers high-quality care, but how could we prove it? Audit provides the mechanism for doing this and is a key element in the clinical governance programmes which PCGs/LHGs are introducing, as well as being part of the revalidation process.

Additionally, because audit is not a closed circle but a continuous process, new standards can be set and re-audits conducted further down the line to demonstrate that good standards are maintained and that poorer standards have been raised.

Who does the audit?

There are three types of audit.

Self-audit

Self-audit is carried out by individual health professionals or a group within the practice who are investigating their own care. The advantage is that team members can decide which topic they wish to investigate and hence the sense of ownership is high. The main disadvantage is that because it is a private affair, collusion may occur and difficult questions may not be asked for fear of rocking the boat both professionally and personally. Hence important changes may be sacrificed for the sake of avoiding disruption.

Peer audit

In this process, colleagues from several practices get together to compare their audit findings in relation to a particular topic. Whereas self-audit addresses the questions: 'What do we do, why do we do it and how well do we do it?', peer-group audit adds the following question: 'Are we as competent as our peers?'

This question opens a new dimension and makes us investigate how others achieve better results and how we might emulate them. Peer-group audit may appear more threatening but colleagues from other practices may have a different mind set and hence be able to offer approaches which we may not have considered. Comparisons need not be threatening, because GPs are usually keen to support and learn from each other. Very often, colleagues from other practices are quicker to find reasons for our shortcomings than we are ourselves!

External audit

External audit differs from those described above because it is conducted by external assessors who are not colleagues, and may not even be (as with lay assessors) from the same profession. They may not, therefore, share the same values and priorities as ourselves.

Examples of external assessment are the Charter Mark awards and the Quality Practice Award, the latter offered by the RCGP. These awards offer the practice an opportunity to compare their standards with those rigorously developed by other agencies, such as our fellow professionals in primary and secondary care, our patients and our employers. There is usually no scope for arguing with the criteria that have to be met, and only if we believe these criteria to be valid is the commitment worth undertaking.

Assessments of this type also take a global view of how the practice functions. This means that not only are the separate components of healthcare examined, but also how well they fit together. There is a point to this, because unless team members are competent and the organisation fairly seamless, the best-quality clinical care cannot be delivered. Such a wide-ranging audit is not within the scope of self-audit or peer-group audit and is a potential advantage of submitting ourselves to external assessors.

External assessment is the most daunting prospect of those described, but the potential gains are also the greatest, resulting in improved self-esteem, better team working and an enhanced reputation for the practice, justified because of the higher standards of care being delivered.

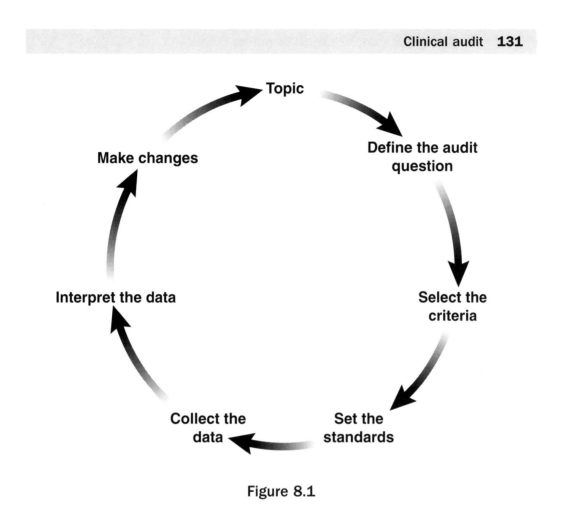

Figure 8.1

How do I conduct an audit?

Conducting an audit means undertaking a process which is best thought of as being ongoing, and is illustrated in Figure 8.1.

Choose a topic

The first thing to decide is what to audit. An appropriate subject should be one which:

- *Is important*: meaning that it is a clinical area which, if managed well, is likely to have significant benefits for the patients and the practice, or may have significant adverse consequences if managed poorly. When choosing a topic we might ask ourselves:

– In which areas of care do we have concerns regarding our performance?

– Which areas of care are being prioritised by the profession and society generally?

– In which areas have there recently been significant advances, for example therapeutically, in primary care management?

• *Has feasibility for improvement*: i.e. that there are interventions which would improve on our current patient management, and the expertise and resources to make use of the interventions available.

• *Is measurable*: meaning that with relation to the topic being studied, there are elements that not only define performance, but can be measured reliably. Hence we might be able to audit the diagnosis of depression through retrospective case analysis, the use of a depression inventory, etc., but we might find it almost impossible to audit the quality of counselling offered to our patients.

Define the audit question

Having decided on the general topic area (e.g. cardiac failure) we need to narrow this down to a specific audit question (for example, 'Do we assess patients for ACEI treatment in line with locally agreed guidelines?').

The purpose of doing this is that it allows us to set the criteria appropriately and specifically in line with the question we wish to answer. It also prevents us from asking too broad a question which runs the risk of being unanswerable, leading to time being wasted and the process of audit acquiring a negative reputation.

Selecting the criteria

The criteria are, quite simply, those items related to the audit question which can be measured or objectively assessed. Wherever possible the criteria should be evidence-based, or at the very least, capable of being justified. Thus in the example on the use of ACEIs in cardiac failure, one criterion that we could choose which is both measurable and justifiable might be: 'Before commencing ACEIs, the patient's suspected cardiac failure should be confirmed by echocardiography.

Setting standards

When we define a criterion, it should be capable of having a standard attached, hence the importance of having an evidence-base from which to decide what that standard should be.

Very rarely is a standard of 100% appropriate in practice. We may initially wish to conduct an audit without setting a standard in order to establish a baseline. This is a practical approach that avoids us becoming disillusioned or overconfident if our initial standard was inappropriately high or low. Usually, we try to set an *optimal* standard which is derived from a combination of:

- what the literature tells us represents good practice
- the implications of falling short of a gold standard
- what we know to be feasible given our resources and the communities we serve.

Thus for our heart failure patients, we may choose to accept a standard of 70% of them to be assessed by echocardiography, because there are restrictions on the availability of the procedure and because there are other methods of diagnosing heart failure. However, we would not be prepared to accept the same figure as the standard for knowing the rubella antibody status in the female population at risk from congenital rubella syndrome, because of the catastrophic nature of this preventable condition.

Collecting the data

This can be collected from various sources such as reviewing the patients' notes, prospective data gathering, PACT data, and the use of questionnaires and interviews. When patient numbers are small, e.g. fewer than 50, the aim is to collect a complete data set. With larger numbers, a random sampling method such as examining every fifth record could be chosen.

Interpreting the data

The object is to keep any analysis as simple as possible. Thus we may present the data in tabular form or perhaps as a graph or histogram, but formal statistical analysis should not be needed.

The purpose of interpretation is to answer the question 'Have we reached the performance standard or not?'. If the standard has been reached, we should double-check that we didn't set the standard too low, and also ask ourselves what the concern was that prompted the initial inquiry. Might it have been that the criteria we chose were inappropriate and could not have addressed the initial question in the way we thought that they would?

If, as is usually the case, we have not attained the standard then the discussion should move on to consider the reasons why.

The way that the audit results are fed back needs careful thought. With clinical audit it is important that doctors can see how their performance compares with that of their colleagues, as this may be a significant motivator for change. To minimise the risk of embarrassment and loss of esteem, each doctor could be presented with a sheet of anonymised data showing comparisons between doctors. The person presenting the audit could maintain confidentiality by only allowing individuals to know which set of data refers to them, although admittedly this technique does not work in two-handed practices!

Some doctors are less reserved and are willing to compare themselves more openly. Once doctors become more familiar with audit, this approach works better because it allows for a more fruitful discussion of why differences occur and how improvements can be made.

Making changes

Once we have swallowed our pride and recognised that there is room for improvement we should turn our attention to how this might be achieved. It may be the case that in order to reach the audit standard, improvement is only required of isolated individuals, in which case the changes needed can be addressed by these individuals through their PDPs. More often, however, the improvements required are more generalised, involving several people and affecting the management of clinical care as well as its content.

In these situations, we must first decide whether the changes needed to achieve the improvement are worth the effort expended. We have only limited resources (meaning time, finances and energy) and therefore there should be consensus when the priorities for the practice are chosen. The changes proposed must be feasible and equitable for all concerned. Hence it might be inappropriate for a partner who seldom performs gynaecological examinations to insist that his colleagues opportunistically screen for chlamydia using cervical swabs.

Review of the topic

Having decided on the changes we wish to implement, we set new standards which will be more realistic and probably higher than the first time round, and conduct a further audit. This process, which allows us to check whether agreed changes are being implemented, is called completing the audit cycle or 'closing the loop'.

Continuous monitoring

When audits are repeated, they are done periodically, usually after a set interval. Nowadays, with the increasing sophistication of practice computers, there are electronic systems which allow for continuous monitoring of various parameters either pre-programmed in the software or set by the practice.

Continuous monitoring not only allows important areas of care to be kept under surveillance, such as glycosylated Hb in diabetics, but allows trends to be recognised and, where necessary, corrective action to be taken before a problem develops. Continuous monitoring helps us to look at our individual performance, the management of individual patients and also the healthcare delivered to larger groups.

Who can help me?

Audit departments (Primary Care Audit Groups and MAAGs) are established in every health authority, and their personnel can advise about how to conduct audits and interpret them. Additionally, they have information relating to other audits conducted on similar topics and on audit activity in your area.

Information is also available to enable practices to compare data with each other. Clinical governance departments have a responsibility to collate audit details of practices within their PCGs and these data may be available in some form for your use.

Clinical directorates in secondary care are supported by audit workers who are often willing to help GPs with information and provide assistance with audits, particularly relating to topics which interface with secondary care, such as asthma admissions.

Summary

Unlike significant events, which demand our attention, audit is less dramatic in that it does not proclaim its importance and brings its rewards over a longer timescale. It is nevertheless a powerful method by which to plan and monitor improvements in care and so valuable is it considered to be, that audit activity is likely to form part of the requirement for Revalidation. Most GPs are perpetually interested in their work and in the standards which their practices achieve, and audit is a natural extension of this interest. When audit is unsuccessful, it is usually because the audit question was too big, but provided the question is clearly focused and the audit cycle is followed, the experience of audit should be a positive and useful one.

When engaging in audit for the first time, GPs are often surprised as to how simple it is, but as we have seen throughout this book, nearly all the techniques we use to further our education are straightforward and within everyone's grasp.

9 The future of PDPs

Introduction

What are PPDPs?

How can they help us?

How can our PPDP be developed?

Example of producing an in-house PPDP

Using an external framework

Summary

Further information

Key points

- PDPs are personal, but will in future need to take account of the needs of the practice.
- When the healthcare team uses a PPDP, it needs first to define the practice goals.
- Goals reflect the team's needs and wants and may be informed by influences outside the practice.
- These goals are met by task forces drawn from the whole team.
- The skills that those in the task forces require will signpost their learning needs.
- Individuals can incorporate these learning needs in their PDPs.
- Only a few of an individual's learning needs will be dictated by the needs of the practice.
- PPDPs encourage teams to plan together, learn together and achieve together.
- This means that although GPs may have a lead role, they no longer have sole responsibility for meeting the practice's targets.

Introduction

Times are changing fast and for many GPs moving from the educational system of the past to the challenges (and potential) of PDPs, will be enough of a cultural shift to contend with. Why then should we consider practice professional development plans (PPDPs), thereby introducing a further complication and another awful acronym? The reason is that General Medical Services are provided by teams, and the goals that we aspire to and are required to meet can only be achieved by good team working. To meet these goals, members of the team must have the appropriate skills, which in turn means that they will have certain educational requirements. The PPDP, by defining the goals and mapping out the training and educational requirements of the team in relation to these, helps to make our learning effective and therefore our goals attainable.

What are PPDPs?

In 1998, the then Chief Medical Officer, Kenneth Calman, started serious consideration of these plans through his recommendation 'to integrate and improve the educational process through the Practice Professional Development Plan, developing the concept of the whole team'. The idea is that members of the primary healthcare team should stop working on their professional development in isolation from each other. Instead, in recognition of the fact that we are all aiming for the same target of improved patient care, we should join forces in developing a plan. This plan should define the practice goals, those who will take responsibility for the areas identified, and the educational requirements that they might have as a result. Unlike our PDP, which may be written annually, the PPDP may describe a strategy over a longer period. Figure 9.1 illustrates the process, which is further explained later in this chapter.

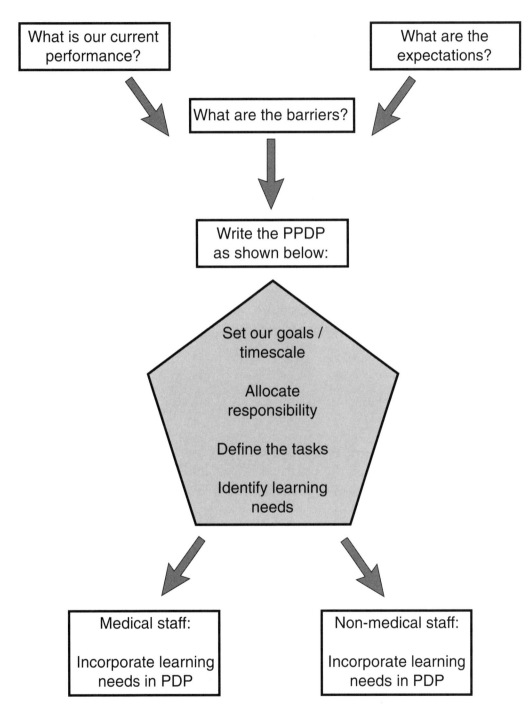

Figure 9.1 The PPDP: where it fits in.

How can they help us?

The first rule of education is to create the need, so even if a PPDP is not compulsory, why should we think seriously about having one? Here are a few reasons.

Developing an effective team

Although many GPs consider themselves to be part of a primary healthcare team, how well developed, coherent and effective are our teams in reality? We may know the channels of communication and exchange information with each other, and we will certainly have defined the roles and responsibilities and the mechanisms of accountability. However, to what degree do we achieve the following:

- set time aside to meet with each other?
- empower colleagues to define the values and goals of the team?
- encourage all members of the team to share their experiences and learn from each other?
- encourage team members to succeed by providing support and by rewarding achievement?

These attributes are characteristic of practice teams that have flattened their hierarchy, meaning not that the roles and responsibilities have changed, but that team members are encouraged to understand and value each other's contribution and to regard each other more as equals. Such teams are sometimes called 'learning organisations' which implies that they are both *organised* with good practice management, policies and protocols, and that they have *mechanisms for learning* from each other.

In the modern NHS, effective teams are synonymous with learning organisations and the PPDP can help us to develop those attributes listed above because it requires us to:

- create the need in the team for the PPDP, by encouraging everyone to recognise that we have common goals, we need education to achieve those goals and that education is a joint responsibility
- protect time for developing the PPDP

- obtain representation from all members of the team
- encourage contribution from all members in setting goals. This is often a turning point in team development, as it may be the first time that some members (e.g. receptionists) have been asked to say where they think the strengths and weaknesses of the practice lie, and how the practice could move forward. The value of encouraging people to feel that they have a voice that others want to hear cannot be overstated
- delegate responsibility for achieving these goals to task groups. These groups, which will nearly always be multidisciplinary, will have a lead member who can be *anyone* from the team, with the others acting in a support role. The groups will not only bring about improvements in patient care, but by ensuring that the systems on which these improvements are based are in place, they will also improve the organisation of the practice
- identify the learning needs of these groups using some of the techniques discussed earlier in this book, and decide how these needs can be met
- encourage team members to include these learning needs in their own PDPs
- create a mechanism for the sharing of information and learning with the rest of the team.

Improving team development

In order to develop, members of the team first need to understand each other. They may have some knowledge of each other's roles and responsibilities but in the early stages even this should not be taken for granted. Knowing what your colleague does is one step closer to understanding what motivates them and what their values and aspirations are, but appreciating this 'culture' can be difficult to do directly. For GPs and their teams a particularly good way of coming to understand each other is to work together, and the PPDP is an ideal way of doing this. This is because the task groups are multidisciplinary, have common goals, have responsibilities to each other and the wider team, and have protected time for this purpose. Most important, the usual power brokers of the practice may not occupy a lead role, and the group works on the basis of an equal partnership.

It is a common experience among members of these groups that the gains made in mutual understanding are at least as great as the stated goals which the groups were set up to achieve.

As understanding develops, team members become both more tolerant and helpful to each other and more willing to broaden their own horizons, taking an interest in activities which they did not previously see as being within their remit.

Improving clinical care

If there was ever a time when conscientious and competent GPs could achieve high standards of patient care independently of their colleagues, that time has long since passed. Nowadays, more can be done and more people have a role to play. For example, in the prevention of coronary heart disease GPs will be brushing up on the management of hypertension and the prescribing of statins; practice nurses will be involved in multiple risk factor assessment; the health visitors with smoking cessation advice; and the receptionists with patient information leaflets and advice on services.

Increasingly, our political masters and the public want to see improved patient outcomes as a result of our training and education. As family doctors we want this too, and the PPDP allows us to state an outcome for, say, the secondary prevention of coronary heart disease, and plan the training of those involved in meeting this goal. We may not be able to guarantee that the goal will be achieved, but with a system in place it is much more likely that we will succeed and that our patients will benefit.

Planning educational activity

In the past, if some educational event was available which addressed a practice need, it was more by accident than design. The PPDP allows us to determine our educational requirements and seek advice as to how these can be met. Quite often our needs will be similar to those of other practices, especially when national targets are involved, and the clinical governance groups will help to organise suitable training. At other times our needs may be practice-specific in which case education tutors can advise us to the available options.

While team members will still go to lectures, attend courses and take study leave, because the PPDP defines educational needs common to several members of the team, much more of our learning will be in-house. Such practice-based learning is both more useful and more convenient – the era when we no longer have to rush back from a meeting in order to start a surgery or clinic, or waste hours trying to park a car can't come too soon!

Improving corporate planning

The phrase 'corporate planning' may sound alien to most GPs, but we are increasingly finding that the techniques and systems we use and adopt are commonplace in industry. Most GPs have business plans or practice development plans that are used to plan for what we think the future might bring. Our PPDP makes us think about the services we wish to provide and consider not only the educational needs but also the resource implications in terms of manpower, equipment, space and so on. The PPDP also allows us to be less reactive and more proactive in terms of deciding our priorities. National targets, and hopefully local ones, should have feasible timescales and if incorporated into the PPDP there is a better chance that they can be achieved without the trauma of a last-minute crisis. This is an important factor in maximising the educational benefit of these initiatives.

Business plans are needed to ensure the viability of the practice; PPDPs are needed to define the clinical direction of the practice and the resources that this requires. Each plan is heavily influenced by the other and in order to organise effectively for the future, it is sensible to have both.

Providing a mechanism of accountability

PPDPs aid accountability at two levels – within the practice it defines who is responsible for achieving what and over what timescale; for external agencies, particularly those concerned with clinical governance, the PPDP is proof that we have a framework in place to deliver our targets and attend to the professional development of our teams.

Helping to bid for resources

Bidding for resources is much more likely to be successful if we have objective proof such as a PPDP to demonstrate that our needs have been carefully considered, and that our requirements have been defined by the whole team. With regard to the future, if we fail to meet the set targets, documentary proof of genuine underfunding is an important defence against criticism.

How can our PPDP be developed?

Let us consider this by referring back to Figure 9.1. Various approaches are being developed and this is but one model, although the principles described will be common to many.

Preparatory work

The first stage is to ensure that time is put aside, people understand the purpose and clear objectives are established. We will not consider the nuts and bolts of how to run these meetings as your GP tutor can advise you. The overall aim is to define certain goals that the practice wants to meet and a good starting point is to perform a SWOT analysis in which the team considers the Strengths and Weaknesses of the practice, the Opportunities it has and the perceived Threats to its development.

The first objective is to encourage team members to establish the *current performance* of the practice. They can do this by asking such questions as:

- what are the strengths of the practice? What does it do well? What are its successes?
- how does it perform in comparison to other practices? We might look at the results of audits, PACT data, referrals, etc
- what is its level of organisation? Are practice policies and protocols kept up to date? Are they accessible? Are they implemented?
- what are the weaknesses of the practice? What about the standard of the premises, accessibility and range of services, patient complaints, concerns of the staff, etc?

Next we can think about the *expectations*, both those that others have of us and those ambitions that we have for the practice. The stakeholders in our services are the people and organisations who employ and regulate us, as well as those who use our services. The former group usually tells us what they require such as meeting National Service Framework guidelines, but how clear are we about the needs of our patients? Do we ask?

Our own expectations may derive from personal ambitions, such as becoming a GP trainer, or the recognition of opportunities, such as the purchase of a new computer which makes the paperless practice a possibility. We may wish to commit ourselves to external review in which our goals are laid down for us – we consider this in the next section.

Remember that we are not yet considering the feasibility of these suggestions and therefore it is appropriate at this point for team members to state what they *hope* for, or what the characteristics of our ideal practice might be. This might include suggestions about the types of personnel (e.g. nurse practitioner) and standards of training as well as types of service. If all this seems like pie-in-the-sky we should remember one thing – if we don't ask, we will never get!

Back to Earth now, with a consideration of the *barriers*. The team might highlight human factors such as a lack of will or commitment; structural factors such as a lack of adequate premises or information technology; financial factors such as a lack of resources to purchase equipment or employ staff and so on.

Writing the PPDP

Putting these considerations together, the team is now in a position to make some choices and everyone should be involved in brainstorming the possible goals and then prioritising these. Bearing in mind that some of these goals will be long term, ownership of them is vital to maintaining the interest of the team and their motivation. It is also important that the goals chosen should be feasible, which means that the barriers identified should not be insuperable.

We next have to decide who will take responsibility for achieving the goals. A co-ordinator will be needed to oversee the process and ensure that the goals are achieved on time – this person might well be the practice manager. The people assigned to each goal should have an interest as well as a responsibility in that area, and be encouraged to feel that they have something to contribute. For each goal, a named person will take the lead role and a small group of others will support the lead.

Each goal should then be divided into a series of tasks that when undertaken result in the goal being achieved – rather like the way we saw in Chapter 3 (that meeting our educational objectives will result in our learning aim being achieved). Begin dividing goals into broad tasks by using suggestions from the whole team, which can be later refined by the responsible group.

When the tasks are defined, it is then possible to allocate particular tasks to individuals or small groups of individuals. At this point the individuals concerned should ask themselves if they have the necessary knowledge or skills to complete these tasks – if not, they will have identified learning needs that must be addressed.

Attending to learning needs

The mechanism for doing this is for individuals to incorporate these needs in their PDPs. In Figure 9.1, the learning needs that arise from the PPDP are split artificially between medical and non-medical staff. This emphasises that training and educational needs are as relevant to non-medical personnel as they are to doctors and nurses.

Example of producing an in-house PPDP

In the example that follows, one goal is identified and developed. A PPDP is a collection of a few such goals developed in a similar manner.

Background
The practice was concerned to develop a smoking cessation strategy.

Current performance
- This was derived from computer records and showed that while smoking status was recorded for over 70% of patients, for many patients the data was over five years old.
- Smokers had often not been followed up and no computer record existed regarding any advice given.

Expectations
- The NHS smoking cessation programme makes it clear that healthcare professionals should question patients at every opportunity regarding smoking status, establish their readiness to quit and offer appropriate support.
- Members of the team also felt strongly that this important factor in coronary heart disease prevention should be tackled vigorously.
- Increasing numbers of smokers were asking for help, particularly with regard to nicotine replacement therapy.

Barriers
- Education was identified as a barrier, with uncertainty regarding what advice to give.
- Lack of resources to offer more detailed advice and support.
- Ignorance of how to enter data regarding smoking status/advice onto the new computer system.

Writing the PPDP
The goals, tasks, personnel involved and their learning needs were identified and written in the PPDP – *see* table [p. 148].

A PPDP template for your use is included at the end of this chapter.

Using an external framework

As we have seen, there are many factors that influence the goals we choose for our PPDP. Only one factor is unchanging, i.e. compulsory targets are compulsory and

Practice professional development plan
Goal: To develop a smoking cessation strategy for the practice

Name	Position	Role	Task	Learning need/method
Margaret Foster	Health visitor	Lead	Provide smoking cessation counselling Establish support group	Attend course for cessation counsellors
Gargi Kalsi	GP	Support	Formulate advice to be offered in consultation Produce patient information leaflet	Read national guidelines for health professionals
Wendy Heath	Practice nurse	Support	Produce protocol regarding advice offered in clinic and the referral pathway	Develop protocol with colleagues in practice nurse forum
John Glossop	Computer operator	Support	Teach medical staff how to quickly enter and update data	Obtain training on Read codes, establishing template and a system to prompt updates

should therefore be included in our plan. But where do we go from here? To decide which other goals are appropriate we need guidance as to which standards define 'good practice', and this is where an external framework such as the RCGP *Quality Practice Award* or the King's Fund *Commitment to Quality* programme can be useful.

These programmes help us to achieve good practice and become learning organisations through improving communication at all levels of the practice, promoting a culture of sharing, and encouraging us to make a public statement on the quality of our services. Unlike the situation of 'going it alone', participating in these programmes brings valuable support both from the organisers and from other practices who are taking part or have done so before. In addition, funding is sometimes available for those who participate.

Although the practices that have taken part in such schemes have traditionally been the highly organised types who seem to have had practice managers for the past 50 years, the ones that gain most from these programmes are the novices. With PPDPs just around the corner, now is a good time to look at the criteria of such schemes. Your PCG/LHG will advise you as to which ones are being used locally and you can find out more about the RCGP and King's Fund programmes at the end of this chapter.

Even if the practice decides not to commit itself to such a scheme, the criteria map out the range of areas in which a practice should seek to be competent. This is a useful template for the team to discuss, and can influence the goals we choose. As an example, *Commitment to Quality* describes standards in the following four areas.

Practice management standards:

- annual development plan
- access to services
- involving patients
- information for patients
- complaints
- management of health records
- administrative audit
- child protection

- carers
- information management and technology
- financial management
- health and safety
- security of premises
- premises and equipment
- written procedures
- partnership agreement.

Team development standards:

- recruitment and selection
- induction and orientation
- staffing arrangements
- education and training
- communication and teamwork
- communication and teamwork (nursing team).

Clinical effectiveness standards:

- manual of clinical guidelines
- management of asthma
- management of diabetes
- management of coronary heart disease
- management of a selection from the following: chronic heart failure/ hypertension/stroke prevention/upper GI disorders/epilepsy/back pain/sexually transmitted diseases
- mental health and social care
- management of severe enduring mental illness
- management of drug and alcohol misuse
- management of depression
- management of dementia

- palliative care
- wound care
- continence care
- maternity care
- cervical cytology
- child health promotion and immunisation
- providing appropriate consultation time
- health record content
- referrals
- clinical audit.

Prescribing standards:

- quality of prescribing
- repeat prescribing
- generic prescribing
- management of medicines.

No matter how well developed our practices are, this list will seem intimidating. However, many frameworks are more concerned with having *systems* in place and leave such things as organisational or clinical standards to be decided on by the practice. On the next page is an example from *Commitment to Quality* – as you can see, the indicators are sensible and allow us to set standards according to what *we* think is achievable.

Practice Management Standard No. 2: Access to services

Quality indicators:
- the telephone system is appropriate for the needs of patients and staff and is reviewed at least every two years
- the team has guidelines for the length of wait for routine appointments and clear procedures for emergency access
- patients are able to access care through no more than two phone calls
- the team has written guidelines for home visits
- the team has clear procedures for contacting staff on duty or away from the premises, which includes message management
- the team has clear procedures for processing repeat prescriptions
- the practice has a clear procedure for responding to patient enquiries.

Having an overview may also bring to mind areas that we have not considered or have persistently chosen to overlook! For example, under 'health and safety' we may have considered how to dispose of 'sharps' but may not have determined the Hepatitis B status of our staff. Alternatively, under 'education and training' we may realise that it has been some time since the receptionists received training in basic life-support skills.

How then do criteria such as these fit in with our PPDP? It is important to remember that programmes such as *Commitment to Quality* do not in themselves constitute our professional development plan. What they do is provide goals that we can choose to commit ourselves to in whole, in part or not at all. To produce our PPDP we still need to translate our goals, from whatever source, into allocated tasks and determine the training and education implications of these tasks, as shown earlier.

Summary

This book has been about the future of GP education. The Bristol inquiry and the Shipman case are two of the blackest clouds ever to pass over medicine's face, but we don't have to look too closely to see a silver lining. In the end, the profession, the public and the politicians all want the same thing, which is a system to ensure that good standards of patient care are maintained – and to achieve this, high-quality postgraduate education has become a national priority. We have seen how the PDP will liberate us from the constraints of PGEA, and learned a good deal about the techniques by which our learning needs can be disclosed and attended to. With the PPDP, we have also seen how GPs will no longer have to take sole responsibility for maintaining and developing the quality of the practice. It is clear that the PPDP could, over a period of time, empower and motivate our teams in a way that we have not previously experienced, leading to enhanced job satisfaction all-round. The future is about taking joint responsibility for developing the practice and for learning together. For GPs, enjoying learning as we do, the prospect of reducing our chores and increasing our pleasures must surely be a welcome one.

Further information

- *Commitment to Quality*: a development of the King's Fund Organisational Audit.

  Details from:

  CTQ Co-ordinator
  Sheffield Health
  5 Old Fulwood Road
  Sheffield
  S10 3TG

- *Quality Practice Award*

  Details from RCGP web-site: www.rcgp.org.uk

- *The TVF (Team, Vision, Future) Workshops*: a pioneering and practical approach to developing PPDPs through a series of facilitated meetings.

  Details from:

  Dr Safiy Karim
  Adviser in Postgraduate GP Education
  Postgraduate Centre
  Queen's Medical Centre
  Nottingham
  NG7 2UH

- Irvine D and Irvine S (1996) *The Practice of Quality*. Radcliffe Medical Press. (Out of print.)

  A prophetic and practical book, this text examines how practices can deliver quality through effective teamwork, sound management and sharing their learning experiences.

- Pendleton D and Hasler J (1997) *Professional Development in General Practice*. Oxford Medical Publications, Oxford.

  With contributions from several leading GP educationists, this book is a thought-provoking overview of several mechanisms which can be used to further our professional development, including learning consultation skills and the use of practice visits, facilitators and mentoring.

Practice professional development plan
Goal:

Name	Position	Role	Task	Learning need/method

Further information

Internet

One good source of audit advice, which also has some impressive audit protocols, is the National Centre for Clinical Audit. They can be contacted through the home page of the National Institute for Clinical Excellence:

www.nice.org.uk

Alternatively, you can write to:

Eli Lilly National Clinical Audit Centre
Department of General Practice
Leicester General Hospital
University of Leicester
Gwendolen Road
Leicester
LE5 4PW

Other Internet sources of information on audits include a variety of audit protocols which can be downloaded:

www.suffolk-maag.ac.uk/disease/index.html

www.equip.ac.uk

www.le.ac.uk/cgrdu

Information on the *Quality Practice Award* and Fellowship by assessment offered by the RCGP, both of which are subject to external assessment, can be obtained from:

www.rcgp.org.uk

Books

Irvine D and Irvine S (1997) *Making Sense of Audit* (2e). Radcliffe Medical Press, Oxford. (Out of print.)

One of the clearest books on the subject with many examples drawn from practice life.

Baker R, Hearnshaw H and Robertson N (eds) (1999) *Implementing Change with Clinical Audit.* John Wiley & Sons, Chichester.

This book looks particularly at the barriers to change and how they might be overcome.

Lawrence M and Schofield T (1993) *Medical Audit in Primary Health Care.* Oxford General Practice Series No. 25. Oxford University Press, Oxford.

A book which gives examples of how audit can be applied to specific areas of general practice.

Grol R and Lawrence M (1995) *Quality Improvement by Peer Review.* Oxford General Practice Series No. 32. Oxford University Press, Oxford.

For those interested in peer group assessment, this book is a practical guide to the process.

Index